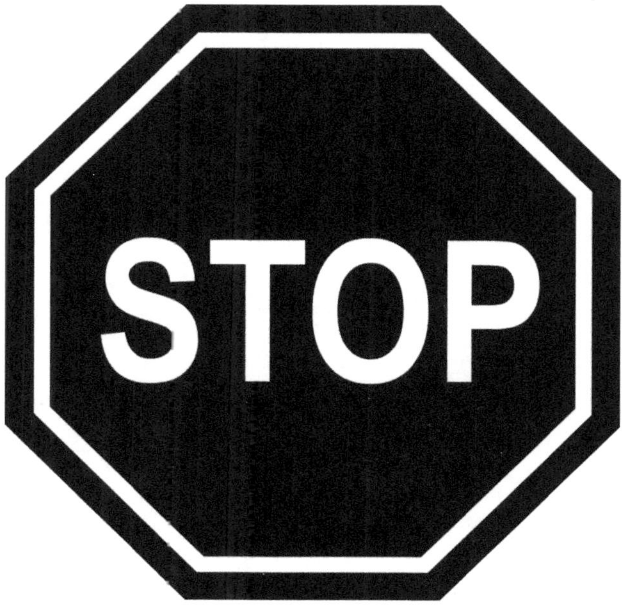

FREE Test Taking Tips Video/DVD Offer

To better serve you, we created videos covering test taking tips that we want to give you for FREE. **These videos cover world-class tips that will help you succeed on your test.**

We just ask that you send us feedback about this product. Please let us know what you thought about it—whether good, bad, or indifferent.

To get your **FREE videos**, you can use the QR code below or email freevideos@studyguideteam.com with "Free Videos" in the subject line and the following information in the body of the email:

a. The title of your product

b. Your product rating on a scale of 1-5, with 5 being the highest

c. Your feedback about the product

If you have any questions or concerns, please don't hesitate to contact us at info@studyguideteam.com.

Thank you!

Test Prep Books

SCAN HERE

CFPN Study Guide

CFPN Exam Prep and Practice Test Questions for the Certified Foundational Perioperative Nurse Test [Includes Detailed Answer Explanations]

Joshua Rueda

Written and edited by TPB Publishing.

ISBN 13: 9781637758649
ISBN 10: 1637758642

Table of Contents

Quick Overview

As you draw closer to taking your exam, effective preparation becomes more and more important. Thankfully, you have this study guide to help you get ready. Use this guide to help keep your studying on track and refer to it often.

This study guide contains several key sections that will help you be successful on your exam. The guide contains tips for what you should do the night before and the day of the test. Also included are test-taking tips. Knowing the right information is not always enough. Many well-prepared test takers struggle with exams. These tips will help equip you to accurately read, assess, and answer test questions.

A large part of the guide is devoted to showing you what content to expect on the exam and to helping you better understand that content. In this guide are practice test questions so that you can see how well you have grasped the content. Then, answer explanations are provided so that you can understand why you missed certain questions.

Don't try to cram the night before you take your exam. This is not a wise strategy for a few reasons. First, your retention of the information will be low. Your time would be better used by reviewing information you already know rather than trying to learn a lot of new information. Second, you will likely become stressed as you try to gain a large amount of knowledge in a short amount of time. Third, you will be depriving yourself of sleep. So be sure to go to bed at a reasonable time the night before. Being well-rested helps you focus and remain calm.

Be sure to eat a substantial breakfast the morning of the exam. If you are taking the exam in the afternoon, be sure to have a good lunch as well. Being hungry is distracting and can make it difficult to focus. You have hopefully spent lots of time preparing for the exam. Don't let an empty stomach get in the way of success!

When travelling to the testing center, leave earlier than needed. That way, you have a buffer in case you experience any delays. This will help you remain calm and will keep you from missing your appointment time at the testing center.

Be sure to pace yourself during the exam. Don't try to rush through the exam. There is no need to risk performing poorly on the exam just so you can leave the testing center early. Allow yourself to use all of the allotted time if needed.

Remain positive while taking the exam even if you feel like you are performing poorly. Thinking about the content you should have mastered will not help you perform better on the exam.

Once the exam is complete, take some time to relax. Even if you feel that you need to take the exam again, you will be well served by some down time before you begin studying again. It's often easier to convince yourself to study if you know that it will come with a reward!

Test-Taking Strategies

1. Predicting the Answer

When you feel confident in your preparation for a multiple-choice test, try predicting the answer before reading the answer choices. This is especially useful on questions that test objective factual knowledge. By predicting the answer before reading the available choices, you eliminate the possibility that you will be distracted or led astray by an incorrect answer choice. You will feel more confident in your selection if you read the question, predict the answer, and then find your prediction among the answer choices. After using this strategy, be sure to still read all of the answer choices carefully and completely. If you feel unprepared, you should not attempt to predict the answers. This would be a waste of time and an opportunity for your mind to wander in the wrong direction.

2. Reading the Whole Question

Too often, test takers scan a multiple-choice question, recognize a few familiar words, and immediately jump to the answer choices. Test authors are aware of this common impatience, and they will sometimes prey upon it. For instance, a test author might subtly turn the question into a negative, or he or she might redirect the focus of the question right at the end. The only way to avoid falling into these traps is to read the entirety of the question carefully before reading the answer choices.

3. Looking for Wrong Answers

Long and complicated multiple-choice questions can be intimidating. One way to simplify a difficult multiple-choice question is to eliminate all of the answer choices that are clearly wrong. In most sets of answers, there will be at least one selection that can be dismissed right away. If the test is administered on paper, the test taker could draw a line through it to indicate that it may be ignored; otherwise, the test taker will have to perform this operation mentally or on scratch paper. In either case, once the obviously incorrect answers have been eliminated, the remaining choices may be considered. Sometimes identifying the clearly wrong answers will give the test taker some information about the correct answer. For instance, if one of the remaining answer choices is a direct opposite of one of the eliminated answer choices, it may well be the correct answer. The opposite of obviously wrong is obviously right! Of course, this is not always the case. Some answers are obviously incorrect simply because they are irrelevant to the question being asked. Still, identifying and eliminating some incorrect answer choices is a good way to simplify a multiple-choice question.

4. Don't Overanalyze

Anxious test takers often overanalyze questions. When you are nervous, your brain will often run wild, causing you to make associations and discover clues that don't actually exist. If you feel that this may be a problem for you, do whatever you can to slow down during the test. Try taking a deep breath or counting to ten. As you read and consider the question, restrict yourself to the particular words used by the author. Avoid thought tangents about what the author *really* meant, or what he or she was *trying* to say. The only things that matter on a multiple-choice test are the words that are actually in the question. You must avoid reading too much into a multiple-choice question, or supposing that the writer meant something other than what he or she wrote.

5. No Need for Panic

It is wise to learn as many strategies as possible before taking a multiple-choice test, but it is likely that you will come across a few questions for which you simply don't know the answer. In this situation, avoid panicking. Because most multiple-choice tests include dozens of questions, the relative value of a single wrong answer is small. As much as possible, you should compartmentalize each question on a multiple-choice test. In other words, you should not allow your feelings about one question to affect your success on the others. When you find a question that you either don't understand or don't know how to answer, just take a deep breath and do your best. Read the entire question slowly and carefully. Try rephrasing the question a couple of different ways. Then, read all of the answer choices carefully. After eliminating obviously wrong answers, make a selection and move on to the next question.

6. Confusing Answer Choices

When working on a difficult multiple-choice question, there may be a tendency to focus on the answer choices that are the easiest to understand. Many people, whether consciously or not, gravitate to the answer choices that require the least concentration, knowledge, and memory. This is a mistake. When you come across an answer choice that is confusing, you should give it extra attention. A question might be confusing because you do not know the subject matter to which it refers. If this is the case, don't eliminate the answer before you have affirmatively settled on another. When you come across an answer choice of this type, set it aside as you look at the remaining choices. If you can confidently assert that one of the other choices is correct, you can leave the confusing answer aside. Otherwise, you will need to take a moment to try to better understand the confusing answer choice. Rephrasing is one way to tease out the sense of a confusing answer choice.

7. Your First Instinct

Many people struggle with multiple-choice tests because they overthink the questions. If you have studied sufficiently for the test, you should be prepared to trust your first instinct once you have carefully and completely read the question and all of the answer choices. There is a great deal of research suggesting that the mind can come to the correct conclusion very quickly once it has obtained all of the relevant information. At times, it may seem to you as if your intuition is working faster even than your reasoning mind. This may in fact be true. The knowledge you obtain while studying may be retrieved from your subconscious before you have a chance to work out the associations that support it. Verify your instinct by working out the reasons that it should be trusted.

8. Key Words

Many test takers struggle with multiple-choice questions because they have poor reading comprehension skills. Quickly reading and understanding a multiple-choice question requires a mixture of skill and experience. To help with this, try jotting down a few key words and phrases on a piece of scrap paper. Doing this concentrates the process of reading and forces the mind to weigh the relative importance of the question's parts. In selecting words and phrases to write down, the test taker thinks about the question more deeply and carefully. This is especially true for multiple-choice questions that are preceded by a long prompt.

9. Subtle Negatives

One of the oldest tricks in the multiple-choice test writer's book is to subtly reverse the meaning of a question with a word like *not* or *except*. If you are not paying attention to each word in the question, you can easily be led astray by this trick. For instance, a common question format is, "Which of the following is...?" Obviously, if the question instead is, "Which of the following is not...?," then the answer will be quite different. Even worse, the test makers are aware of the potential for this mistake and will include one answer choice that would be correct if the question were not negated or reversed. A test taker who misses the reversal will find what he or she believes to be a correct answer and will be so confident that he or she will fail to reread the question and discover the original error. The only way to avoid this is to practice a wide variety of multiple-choice questions and to pay close attention to each and every word.

10. Reading Every Answer Choice

It may seem obvious, but you should always read every one of the answer choices! Too many test takers fall into the habit of scanning the question and assuming that they understand the question because they recognize a few key words. From there, they pick the first answer choice that answers the question they believe they have read. Test takers who read all of the answer choices might discover that one of the latter answer choices is actually *more* correct. Moreover, reading all of the answer choices can remind you of facts related to the question that can help you arrive at the correct answer. Sometimes, a misstatement or incorrect detail in one of the latter answer choices will trigger your memory of the subject and will enable you to find the right answer. Failing to read all of the answer choices is like not reading all of the items on a restaurant menu: you might miss out on the perfect choice.

11. Spot the Hedges

One of the keys to success on multiple-choice tests is paying close attention to every word. This is never truer than with words like almost, most, some, and sometimes. These words are called "hedges" because they indicate that a statement is not totally true or not true in every place and time. An absolute statement will contain no hedges, but in many subjects, the answers are not always straightforward or absolute. There are always exceptions to the rules in these subjects. For this reason, you should favor those multiple-choice questions that contain hedging language. The presence of qualifying words indicates that the author is taking special care with their words, which is certainly important when composing the right answer. After all, there are many ways to be wrong, but there is only one way to be right! For this reason, it is wise to avoid answers that are absolute when taking a multiple-choice test. An absolute answer is one that says things are either all one way or all another. They often include words like *every*, *always*, *best*, and *never*. If you are taking a multiple-choice test in a subject that doesn't lend itself to absolute answers, be on your guard if you see any of these words.

12. Long Answers

In many subject areas, the answers are not simple. As already mentioned, the right answer often requires hedges. Another common feature of the answers to a complex or subjective question are qualifying clauses, which are groups of words that subtly modify the meaning of the sentence. If the question or answer choice describes a rule to which there are exceptions or the subject matter is complicated, ambiguous, or confusing, the correct answer will require many words in order to be expressed clearly and accurately. In essence, you should not be deterred by answer choices that seem excessively long. Oftentimes, the author of the text will not be able to write the correct answer without offering some qualifications and modifications Your job is to read the answer choices thoroughly and completely and to select the one that most accurately and precisely answers the question.

13. Restating to Understand

Sometimes, a question on a multiple-choice test is difficult not because of what it asks but because of how it is written. If this is the case, restate the question or answer choice in different words. This process serves a couple of important purposes. First, it forces you to concentrate on the core of the question. In order to rephrase the question accurately, you have to understand it well. Rephrasing the question will concentrate your mind on the key words and ideas. Second, it will present the information to your mind in a fresh way. This process may trigger your memory and render some useful scrap of information picked up while studying.

14. True Statements

Sometimes an answer choice will be true in itself, but it does not answer the question. This is one of the main reasons why it is essential to read the question carefully and completely before proceeding to the answer choices. Too often, test takers skip ahead to the answer choices and look for true statements. Having found one of these, they are content to select it without reference to the question above. Obviously, this provides an easy way for test makers to play tricks. The savvy test taker will always read the entire question before turning to the answer choices. Then, having settled on a correct answer choice, he or she will refer to the original question and ensure that the selected answer is relevant. The mistake of choosing a correct-but-irrelevant answer choice is especially common on questions related to specific pieces of objective knowledge. A prepared test taker will have a wealth of factual knowledge at their disposal, and should not be careless in its application.

15. No Patterns

One of the more dangerous ideas that circulates about multiple-choice tests is that the correct answers tend to fall into patterns. These erroneous ideas range from a belief that B and C are the most common right answers, to the idea that an unprepared test-taker should answer "A-B-A-C-A-D-A-B-A." It cannot be emphasized enough that pattern-seeking of this type is exactly the WRONG way to approach a multiple-choice test. To begin with, it is highly unlikely that the test maker will plot the correct answers according to some predetermined pattern. The questions are scrambled and delivered in a random order. Furthermore, even if the test maker was following a pattern in the assignation of correct answers, there is no reason why the test taker would know which pattern he or she was using. Any attempt to discern a pattern in the answer choices is a waste of time and a distraction from the real work of taking the test. A test taker would be much better served by extra preparation before the test than by reliance on a pattern in the answers.

FREE Videos/DVD OFFER

Doing well on your exam requires both knowing the test content and understanding how to use that knowledge to do well on the test. We offer completely FREE test taking tip videos. **These videos cover world-class tips that you can use to succeed on your test.**

To get your **FREE videos**, you can use the QR code below or email freevideos@studyguideteam.com with "Free Videos" in the subject line and the following information in the body of the email:

a. The title of your product

b. Your product rating on a scale of 1-5, with 5 being the highest

c. Your feedback about the product

If you have any questions or concerns, please don't hesitate to contact us at info@studyguideteam.com.

Thanks again!

SCAN HERE

Introduction to the CFPN

Function of the Test

A passing score on the CNOR exam is required to obtain CNOR certification as a registered nurse with the demonstrated knowledge and skills in the field of perioperative nursing. Nurses with CNOR certification are recognized as qualified to provide care to patients before, during, and after surgical procedures. The CNOR certification program is accredited by both of the two major accrediting bodies in nursing: The American Board of Nursing Specialties and the National Commission for Certifying Agencies.

The typical test taker is a registered nurse who wishes to demonstrate mastery in the specialty area of perioperative nursing or nursing duties surrounding a patient's surgical procedure. Licensing demonstrates minimal competence, but CNOR certification shows proficiency, and is intended to enhance professional credibility, demonstrate commitment to the profession, and open doors to promotions and increased compensation. The test is administered throughout the world, but is used primarily in the United States.

Test Administration

Individuals wishing to become CNOR-certified must first apply to take the CNOR test, showing that they 1) hold a current and unrestricted registered nurse license; 2) are working in perioperative nursing; and 3) have completed at least two years and 2,400 hours of work experience in perioperative nursing, with at least 50% of that work in an intraoperative setting.

Once an individual's application is approved, he or she must schedule a test date. The CNOR certification test is offered at Prometric testing centers across the United States. Test takers wishing to take the test outside the United States may do so, and Prometric will do their best to find a testing center within 500 miles of any requested location.

The test is available all year, Monday through Saturday, excluding holidays. However, the test must be taken during a three-month window that begins the month after the test taker's exam application is approved. For example, if a test taker's application is approved in January, he or she must take the exam between February and April or re-apply to take the test at a later date. Individuals wishing to retake the exam may reapply at any time after the close of their testing window. There is no limit on the number of permissible retakes.

In accordance with the Americans with Disabilities Act, individuals with documented disabilities will be provided with appropriate accommodations.

Test Format

Upon arrival at the testing center, test takers must present appropriate identification, such as their driver's license, passport, or military ID, and are then guided to a testing station. Test takers may not bring anything with them into the testing center.

The CNOR test consists of 200 multiple-choice questions, which must be answered in 3 hours and 45 minutes. The questions are delivered via computer and the results are available at the conclusion of the exam.

The content of the CNOR test is intended to assess the candidate's ability to apply their knowledge to the functions and responsibilities of perioperative nurses. It is broken down into the following subject areas:

CNOR Topic Areas	Approx. Percent of Questions
Pre/Postoperative Patient Assessment and Diagnosis	15%
Individualized Plan of Care Development and Expected Outcome	8%
Intraoperative Activities	Patient Care and Safety: 25% Management: 9%
Communication and Documentation	11%
Infection Prevention and Control	16%
Emergency Situations	10%
Professional Accountabilities	6%

Scoring

Test takers receive a raw score that is equal to the number of correct responses. The raw score is then converted to a scaled score between 200 and 800, based on standards intended to equalize each particular form or version of the test. A scaled score of 620 is required to pass.

Test results are reported on a pass-fail basis. The pass rate varies over time but is usually around 70%. In 2015, 4,769 candidates took the CNOR, and 67% passed. Test takers who pass are notified at the end of their exam and receive a passing certificate by mail shortly after the successful exam date. Test takers who fail receive a score report that shows their performance in each subject area; however, the report does not address the test taker's performance on a question-by-question basis.

Recent/Future Developments

The content of the CNOR is regularly updated to keep pace with current practice in the field of perioperative nursing. However, no specific changes to the CNOR's format or structure have been reported recently.

Study Prep Plan for the CFPN Exam

1 **Schedule -** Use one of our study schedules below or come up with one of your own.

2 **Relax -** Test anxiety can hurt even the best students. There are many ways to reduce stress. Find the one that works best for you.

3 **Execute -** Once you have a good plan in place, be sure to stick to it.

One Week Study Schedule

Day 1	Pre/Postoperative Patient Assessment...
Day 2	Intraoperative Activities
Day 3	Communication and Documentation
Day 4	Infection Prevention and Control
Day 5	Emergency Situations
Day 6	Practice Test
Day 7	Take Your Exam!

Two Week Study Schedule

Day 1	Pre/Postoperative Patient Assessment...	Day 8	Documenting Perioperative Education
Day 2	Individualized Plan of Care Development...	Day 9	Infection Prevention and Control
Day 3	Intraoperative Activities	Day 10	Emergency Situations
Day 4	Anesthesia Management	Day 11	Professional Accountabilities
Day 5	Surgical Counts	Day 12	Practice Test
Day 6	Management of Intraoperative Activities	Day 13	Answer Explanations
Day 7	Communication and Documentation	Day 14	Take Your Exam!

One Month Study Schedule

Day 1	Pre/Postoperative Patient Assessment and Diagnosis	Day 11	Proper Patient Positioning	Day 21	Practice Questions
Day 2	Medication Reconciliation	Day 12	Management of Intraoperative Activities	Day 22	Emergency Situations
Day 3	Practice Questions	Day 13	Practice Questions	Day 23	Local Anesthetic Systemic Toxicity (LAST)
Day 4	Individualized Plan of Care Development...	Day 14	Communication and Documentation	Day 24	Practice Questions
Day 5	Legal and Ethical Standards	Day 15	Hand-Off Communication	Day 25	Professional Accountabilities
Day 6	Practice Questions	Day 16	Transfer of Care Documentation and Reporting	Day 26	Interdisciplinary Teams and Professional Organizations
Day 7	Intraoperative Activities	Day 17	Practice Questions	Day 27	Practice Questions
Day 8	Preparation of the Surgical Site	Day 18	Infection Prevention and Control	Day 28	Practice Test
Day 9	Environmental Factors	Day 19	Documentation	Day 29	Answer Explanations
Day 10	Specimen Management	Day 20	Personal Protective Equipment	Day 30	Take Your Exam!

Build your own prep plan by visiting:
testprepbooks.com/prep

Pre/Postoperative Patient Assessment and Diagnosis

In preparing the patient for the operative phase of care, the preoperative nurse completes tasks to promote optimal patient outcomes and patient safety. The following text describes routine preoperative tasks.

- Before treatments, medication administration, or transfer of care, the nurse verifies patient identity using two patient identifiers. This is usually done by reading the patient's identification band and asking the patient to state their name and date of birth.
- The nurse verifies the procedure by asking the patient what surgery is being done and by reading the surgical consent and comparing it to the physician order. The nurse also ensures the surgical site is marked, per Universal Protocol.
- The following steps are taken by the nurse to assess the patient's health status.
    - Data is collected, analyzed, and prioritized. The nurse obtains vital signs, performs a pain assessment, reviews allergies and medication intolerances, analyzes lab values, reviews pertinent medical and surgical history (including current and previous medical conditions and family history), reviews the chart, and verifies NPO status.
    - Verbal and nonverbal communication is done utilizing an age-based competency model. This is done during the patient interview process and physical assessment. The nurse should consider the patient's cultural preferences while formulating the plan of care. A common example of this in the preoperative phase is in the Jehovah's Witnesses community, as these patients may not wish to receive blood or blood products.
    - Medication reconciliation occurs prior to surgery. This includes review of the patient's current medication regimen, also noting the use of herbal remedies, vitamins, and supplements. The nurse also notes use of tobacco, alcohol, caffeine, and recreational drugs.
    - Physical assessment is completed; this includes documentation of impaired skin integrity, mobility limitations, and presence of body piercings or implanted foreign objects.
- After collection and review of data, the nurse formulates patient-specific diagnoses. Nursing diagnoses are formulated based on subjective, objective, and psychosocial assessments. These diagnoses provide the foundation for focused nursing care plans. Additional nursing diagnoses are identified along the care continuum, and the nursing care plans are modified accordingly. The nurse may use nursing diagnoses approved by NANDA and PNDS, for instance.
- The nurse's preoperative patient assessment is documented in the medical record. It should be easily retrievable by the interdisciplinary team in order for optimal patient care to take place. Electronic medical records (EMRs) are effective in providing fast, easy access of the preoperative assessment to all members of the health care team. Documentation of the preoperative assessment is imperative for identification of deviations from baseline assessment.

Confirm Patient Identity and Correct Procedure

The Joint Commission

The Joint Commission (TJC) is an international, independent review entity with the mission of ensuring that healthcare facilities operate by and maintain the highest quality standards for care. They accredit organizations based on a stringent set of standards and monitor accredited facilities on two- or three-year cycles. Safety goals are reviewed, and often revised, annually to reflect the most current research and best practice principles.

Universal Protocol

Universal Protocol, enacted by The Joint Commission (TJC) in 2004, is designed to prevent errors involving wrong procedure, wrong patient, and wrong site surgery. This protocol is divided into three categories: patient identity, site marking, and time-out. During the patient identity phase, the nurse uses two patient identifiers—typically, the patient's name and date of birth. The patient's medical record number may also be used. Prior to entering the operating room, the nurse asks the patient to state their name and date of birth while the nurse views the patient's identification band. The nurse verifies the patient's stated information on the patient's ID band with the surgical consent and other documents, if applicable. Surgical site marking occurs if the procedure involves differentiation of right or left side or multiple structures, such as fingers or toes. The operative surgeon completes this prior to induction of anesthesia, involving the patient in the process.

To promote clarity, the site is marked with either the surgeon's initials or with "yes," depending on the protocol of the surgical institution. Marking the operative site with an "X" can be ambiguous and should be avoided. Site marking is performed with a skin marker that remains visible after skin prep. Also, it should be done as close to the surgical site as possible and be visible after the patient is draped. Immediately prior to the procedure, the surgical time-out is performed. The time-out consists of verification of patient identity, procedure, site, position, and availability of implants (if indicated). This occurs after the patient is prepped and draped and when all team members are engaged. All team members participate in the time-out, and if the case doesn't involve general anesthesia or deep sedation, the patient may participate. Each member of the team has the opportunity to ask questions and address concerns during this time.

Informed Consent

Once the physician performing the procedure explains the procedure, risks and benefits, and alternative treatments and provides opportunity for the patient to ask questions, the consent form may be signed. Types of consents obtained preoperatively are surgical, blood, anesthesia, and photography/video consents. These consent forms may be separate, or they may be combined, depending on the health care facility. For example, consent for blood products may be discussed and included in the **surgical consent** document. The nurse may have the consent form signed by the patient once consent is obtained by the physician. If the patient is eighteen years old or older, capable of decision making, and awake, alert, and oriented, the consent form should be signed by the patient. If the patient is incapable of signing the consent form due to impaired mental status or if the patient is incapacitated, the next of kin or power of attorney (POA) should sign it. Additionally, the consent form must be witnessed by another person; this person is usually another nurse or professional who is employed by the operating facility.

The surgical team may not proceed with a procedure if consent isn't obtained; performing a procedure the patient (or next of kin or POA) hasn't consented to can be considered assault. The exception to this is an emergent procedure, where the physician deems the patient's life or limb is in jeopardy unless the procedure is performed. In emergent situations, consent is not required, but the surgeon must document in the medical record the nature of the case and an explanation as to why consent is bypassed.

Allow Natural Death (AND)

It may be beneficial for nurses to discuss "**allow natural death**" practices and decisions with patients and their families during the perioperative process. "Allow natural death" decisions most commonly take place in instances where a surgery is not successful and the patient experiences an event that leads to full or partial brain or heart failure. These events often lead to patient death or a drastically reduced quality of life (such as prolonged life in a vegetative state). Before surgery, patients and their families can make the decision to allow medical staff to gradually decrease life sustaining measures in order to allow the patient to naturally die in comfort.

Patient Self-Determination (PSDA)

The **Patient Self-Determination Act (PSDA)** is administrative legislature that requires healthcare facilities to inform patients of their medical rights, requires that facilities note before a scheduled surgical procedure if patients have legal documentation relating to advance directives and DNR decisions, and requires that healthcare staff have an understanding of general advance directives and DNR decisions. However, the PSDA is a controversial act. Many critics believe an end-of-life discussion with the attending physician is necessary in order for the patient to make fully informed healthcare decisions; however, this is not part of the PSDA.

It is imperative that the entire surgical team verbally concurs with the time-out, and the procedure may not begin until this happens. The time-out is documented by the nurse and placed in the patient's medical record.

Surgical Safety Checklist

Before induction of anaesthesia

SIGN IN

- ☐ Patient has confirmed
  - identity
  - site
  - procedure
  - consent
- ☐ Site marked/not applicable
- ☐ Anaesthesia safety check completed
- ☐ Pulse oximeter on patient and functioning

Does patient have a:

Known allergy?
- ☐ NO
- ☐ YES

Difficult airway/aspiration risk?
- ☐ NO
- ☐ YES, and equipment/assistance available

Risk of >500 ml blood loss (7 ml/kg in children)?
- ☐ NO
- ☐ YES, and adequate intravenous access and fluids planned

Before skin incision

TIME OUT

- ☐ Confirm all team members have introduced themselves by name and role
- ☐ Surgeon, anaesthesia professional and nurse verbally confirm
  - patient
  - site
  - procedure

Anticipated critical events

- ☐ Surgeon reviews:
  What are the critical or unexpected steps, operative duration, anticipated blood loss
- ☐ Anaesthesia team reviews:
  Are there any patient-specific concerns?
- ☐ Nursing team reviews:
  Has sterility (including indicator results) been confirmed?
  Are there equipment issues or any concerns?

Has antibiotic prophylaxis been given within the last 60 minutes?
- ☐ YES
- ☐ Not applicable

Is essential imaging displayed?
- ☐ YES
- ☐ Not applicable

Before patient leaves operating room

SIGN IN

Nurse verbally confirms with the team:

- ☐ The name of the procedure recorded
- ☐ That instrument, sponge and needle counts are correct (*or not applicable*)
- ☐ How the specimen is labelled (*including patient name*)
- ☐ Whether there are any equipment problems to be addressed
- ☐ Surgeon, anaesthesia professional and nurse review the key concerns for recovery and management of the patient

Relevant Patient Data

The nurse uses multiple techniques in performing the **preoperative health assessment**; these include the patient interview, screening tools to identify potential risk for complications, collection of objective data values, and review of the medical record. During the preoperative period, the nurse's data collection should include vital signs, height and weight, review of allergies, NPO (nothing by mouth) status, current pain assessment, skin integrity, presence of implants and body piercings, presence of tubes (such as drains, chest tubes, urinary catheter, percutaneous endoscopic gastrostomy tube, or nasogastric tube), vascular access catheters, and immobilization devices (cast, surgical boot, sling, etc.).

The patient should understand the importance of NPO for surgery because noncompliance compromises the patient's safety by creating risk for aspiration and a compromised airway. Pain should be assessed preoperatively for patient comfort and also to establish the patient's postoperative pain goal. If skin breakdown is present, this must be documented in the medical record as being present on admission. Skin integrity, including risk for impaired skin integrity, is taken into consideration during surgical positioning. Measures such as extra padding with pillows and foam and use of alternate positioning may be utilized to prevent further impairment of the skin. An alternate type of **electrosurgical unit (ESU)** dispersive electrode may be considered in patients with high risk for skin breakdown.

Physical assessment data, along with a review of medical and surgical history, form a picture of the patient's **health status**. The patient interview provides useful information and can also provide insight into potential issues including anxiety, financial worry, discharge planning needs, and psychosocial issues such as domestic abuse. The nurse should consult with interdisciplinary teams when indicated. Focused assessments may be conducted based on initial assessment findings. Screening tools are standards of care and are utilized in the preoperative assessment. The nurse implements plans based on abnormal screening tool findings. For instance, the patient who scores above the desired score upon Obstructive Sleep Apnea screening is automatically referred to the anesthesiologist for follow-up assessment of respiratory risk during surgery. Abnormal assessment findings must be reported to the physician and documented in the medical record.

Laboratory Results

Senior patients almost always require laboratory screening to determine whether or not chronic disease exists, while most other patients will only require laboratory screening if their physical assessment or medical history shows a risk factor for cardiovascular or respiratory disease. These two types of disease, at any stage, can make surgery of any kind a riskier process for the patient; therefore, preparatory measures allow the medical team to provide the safest treatment. Commonly ordered laboratory tests for these conditions include blood counts, electrolyte counts, glucose tests, electrocardiographs, and chest radiographs.

Perioperative Nursing Data Set (PNDS)

The **perioperative nursing data set (PNDS)** is a quality-driven framework that aims to standardize nursing across an organization. It is utilized before, during, and after surgeries in order provide the safest level of care during transition periods for the patient. PNDS systems also serve as a global data collection and management system for the field of nursing. In order to preserve the highest level of standardization, PNDS systems are almost always part of a software package that also supports electronic medical records for the healthcare organization in which it is utilized. This practice reduces human error when transitioning patients between providers. It also allows for fields to collect specific data without changes made from personnel, essential updates to occur in real time and across all stations, and for clean, relevant data collection.

Preoperative Fasting

Preoperative fasting is a preventive measure taken before surgery in order to reduce procedural complications that may occur from a full stomach (such as regurgitation) and the influence of increased metabolic hormones (such as insulin) in the body. This process involves the patient abstaining from food and water for a pre-determined period of time before a procedure. Current research is inconclusive on the length of preoperative fasting that is most effective, but in practice, patients normally fast for a period of two to eight hours based on age and surgery type.

Pathophysiology

Pathophysiology refers to changes in the body due to a disease process. The patient's history of chronic and acute disease is discovered during the preoperative patient interview and chart review. Understanding the pathophysiology of the patient's disease process (or processes) empowers the nurse to know if assessment findings are congruent with the disease process or if findings are indicative of something else.

For example, if a patient has 2+ pitting edema with a history of CHF, the nurse may suspect the edema is secondary to a CHF exacerbation and investigate further by auscultating lung sounds and consulting with a cardiologist. It is also important for the nurse to consider the pathophysiological processes associated with the patient's scheduled procedure. The nurse should note that although the scheduled procedure may be minor, the patient's diagnosis may be quite serious. If the patient is having a PowerPort insertion, the surgery process is minor. However, the patient may have a diagnosis of stage IV lung cancer, and this is quite serious. Understanding this, the nurse may allow more time for the patient to verbalize feelings and provide emotional support for the patient.

Diagnostic Procedures and Results

The diagnostic procedures performed depend on the planned surgical procedure, patient's history, risk factors, and best practice standards. Examples of diagnostic procedures include computerized axial tomography (CT), electrocardiogram (ECG), hemoglobin and hematocrit, pregnancy test for a female patient of childbearing age, type and screen, international normalized ratio (INR), blood glucose, and chest x-ray. These can be done in various settings, such as a physician's office, laboratory, outpatient clinic, or hospital. If a diagnostic procedure shows a deviation from the patient's baseline, such as an ECG change, more tests may be ordered to clear the patient for surgery. In this example, the patient may undergo a cardiac catheterization to determine cardiac risk for surgery.

At this point, the surgeon and cardiologist discuss risks and benefits based on diagnostic data. Occasionally, diagnostic procedures reveal incidental findings that render a patient ineligible for surgery, such as an abdominal aortic aneurysm. In order for nursing diagnoses and medical plans to be formulated, the results of the diagnostic procedures must be documented in the patient's medical record and reviewed prior to surgery.

Appropriate Health Assessment Techniques

Age Specific

Patient age plays an important role in influencing the overall assessment of a preoperative patient. Of course, detailed medical histories of all patients are obtained; however, specific demographics may require additional information. Pediatric patients, for example, are often assessed in conjunction with information provided by their parents. Parents may need to provide information relating to the pediatric patient's birth, congenital health issues that may or may not have been treated, and the achievement (or lack thereof) of developmental milestones. Senior patients should be assessed for both diagnosed and undiagnosed chronic disease.

Cultural Competence

Culture can be defined as the beliefs, values, and social ways of a particular group. These beliefs are generally passed down from generation to generation and can hold influence over one's thoughts and actions. Culture can be the lens that the person uses to view the world, including health and the need for care. Cultural competence of the healthcare workforce and the healthcare delivery system is increasingly tied to improved client outcomes and quality of care provided. Cultural competence is the ability to provide effective care for patients who come from different cultures. It requires sensitivity and effective communication in both verbal and non-verbal communication. Financial reimbursement for care provided to clients can be negatively affected if there is not a system in place to support the culturally competent delivery of care.

A culturally competent clinical nurse will develop an awareness of, and sensitivity to, their own cultural heritage and recognize how their own values and biases may affect patients. The nurse is expected to do the following:

- Demonstrate comfort with cultural differences
- Know specifics about the cultural groups they work with
- Respect and be aware of the unique needs of specific women, men and children
- Understand that diversity exists within and between cultures
- Try to understand other points of view
- Demonstrate flexibility and tolerance, be nonjudgmental
- Maintain a sense of humor
- Demonstrate a willingness to relinquish control
- Promote cultural practices that are potentially helpful

Nurses are aware that unmet cultural or diversity needs and preferences can adversely affect patient outcomes in much the same way that somatic illness affects outcomes. Therefore, cultural sensitivity is an essential nurse competency. The development of cultural sensitivity and demonstrated appreciation of diversity by nurses is also viewed as a continuum in the Synergy Model. Novice nurses, who are learning to negotiate the institutional environment, may assess the patient's preferences but often continue to provide care that is consistent with their own belief system.

As competent nurses gain life and clinical experience, they actively question patients to learn about and accommodate the traditions and customs of a diverse population, while helping the patient and family to understand the culture of the institution. Expert nurses are able to anticipate the needs of the patient and family by integrating cultural differences into the plan of care whenever possible. All of these nursing interventions work to alleviate the stress related to the acute care environment.

Research indicates that diversity in the workplace strengthens the workgroup by allowing consideration of multiple worldviews and a better understanding of the patient population served by the institution. Multiple viewpoints can also be an advantage in conflict resolution, especially when the conflict is related to diversity issues. The Synergy Model suggests that nurses become more sensitive to diversity issues with experience and that this sensitivity is applicable to the work environment as well as direct patient care. Attention to diversity issues also, however, requires institutional support for resource allocation and management. Depending on the specific needs of the patient population, services such as foreign language interpreters, appropriate food service, counseling services, and accommodation for religious observances must be considered. To optimize patient care, expert nurses assess the needs of the patient and family and provide access to the appropriate institutional resources.

Attention to diversity issues requires that providers proceed on the assumption that ethnocentrism is a universal human characteristic that must be addressed by the provision of appropriate information and instruction. In addition to understanding their own cultural views, nurses must be aware that many patients have preconceived views of western cultural norms, which may or may not be accurate, but can potentially affect the nurse-patient relationship. The resolution of ethnocentrism in a caring relationship requires acknowledgment of its existence and education as to the meaning of the traditions and practices.

Medication Reconciliation

Alcohol Use

At times, a drug may cause an adverse effect when it is co-administered with some other substance that affects its chemical structure or its ability to be absorbed by the body. Narcotics, for example, should not be taken while drinking alcohol. Alcohol, a depressant, exacerbates the effect of the narcotic, also a depressant, to the point that the patient's drive to breathe and their consciousness may be completely knocked out, causing death.

Allergies

Patient **allergies** should always be taken into consideration before any medical procedure. Allergies may affect patient preparation for the procedure, clinical preparation for the procedure, tools and materials used during the procedure, and medications used during recovery.

Contemporary Alternative Medicine (CAM)

Contemporary and alternative medicine (CAM) include health and wellness practices that can occur in tandem to conventional medical care. CAM practices, such as massage, yoga, meditation, acupuncture, and tailored diets often support conventional care or provide a way for patients to manage unpleasant, yet unavoidable, side effects of conventional care. It is important to know if patients engage in CAM modalities, as these should be taken into consideration when preparing for surgical procedures. Additionally, some CAM modalities may be recommended to the patients during the recovery period. It is important to note that not all CAM therapies are evidence-based, as CAM is an emerging field that requires more clinical research.

Herbs

Herbs and herbal medications are a component of CAM, although some conventional practices utilize them (or pharmaceuticals derived from them) as well. Noting whether or not a patient takes any herbal supplements is a vital part of the preoperative process. Many herbal supplements are not regulated by the United States Food and Drug Administration (by standards that conventional pharmaceuticals are); therefore, it is difficult to know what concentration of herbs are actually in these products. Certain levels of common herbal modalities can interfere with anesthetics and other conventional pharmaceuticals, rendering them ineffective or causing unpleasant symptoms in the patient.

Home Meds

In the preoperative phase, the nurse should assess the patient's home medications, which may interfere with anesthesia, intraoperative medications, and postoperative treatments. A full list of home medications should be reconciled to include the name, dosage, frequency, indication, and the last dose taken by the patient. Any medications that are deemed contraindications to the procedure should be promptly reported to the healthcare provider. For example, a patient taking daily warfarin is at a high risk for bleeding. Patients undergoing surgical or invasive procedures would need further considerations from the healthcare provider.

Medical Marijuana

Medical marijuana is an alternative medicine used primarily by patients with chronic pain, anxiety disorders, and altered neuromuscular conditions. Marijuana, or cannabis, is often used recreationally. Many patients may deny its use for fear of judgement. Medical marijuana must be prescribed by a healthcare provider for a specific disease or medical condition. Although prescribed, marijuana used for medical purposes will still exert the same effects as recreational cannabis. The main ingredient in marijuana, delta-9-tetrahydrocannabinol (THC), causes euphoria and decreased coordination while slowing motor activity. The use of medical marijuana may interfere with other prescribed pharmacological treatments and should be included in the medication reconciliation of operative patients.

Medication Reconciliation Protocol

Preoperative review of the current medication regimen is imperative to patient safety and optimal patient outcomes. The **medication reconciliation** process includes a review of all medications, including the name, dosage, route, frequency, and last dose taken. All medications should be recorded; this includes prescription and over-the-counter medications, as well as vitamins, supplements, and herbal remedies. Use of alcohol, tobacco, caffeine, and recreational drugs should also be documented. This information can be obtained through patient and/or family recall or the medication administration record if the patient is from a health care facility. The medication reconciliation should be reviewed by the surgeon and anesthesiologist preoperatively. If certain medications are not stopped prior to the procedure, the surgery may not proceed as planned. For example, if a patient was instructed to stop Plavix seven days prior to the procedure and the medication reconciliation process revealed the patient took Plavix yesterday, the surgeon may deem the surgery unsafe for the patient at this time.

Pharmacology

The nurse should review the **pharmacology**, or the action created by a drug, of the patient's current medications. Knowing the pharmacological effects of these medications and those of the scheduled preoperative medications can help keep the patient safe. If the patient is hypotensive and bradycardic and scheduled to receive a beta-blocker drug as a standing preoperative order, the nurse, understanding the potential pharmacological effects of the beta-blocker, would know to hold the drug and consult the physician. The nurse should have access to online drug references and the capability of consulting with a pharmacist, if needed.

Preoperative Medications

Patients are often prescribed preoperative medications to prevent pain, decrease anxiety, and manipulate gastrointestinal effects. Commonly ordered medications include sedatives such as lorazepam. These medications decrease anxiety and prevent patients from having a recollection of the surgical experience. Narcotics, such as fentanyl or morphine, help with the patient's sedation and can decrease the amount of anesthetic agent needed during the procedure. Anticholinergic medications, such as atropine, decrease respiratory secretions and prevent laryngospasms. Gastric acid production and acidity can be decreased by histamine-2 receptor blockers, such as ranitidine. These medications prevent side effects such as regurgitation and vomiting.

Side Effects of Recreational Drug Use

Nurses must assess a patient's use of recreational drugs during the preoperative assessment. Illicit drugs may cause interactions with the anesthetic agents and alter the effects of intraoperative or postoperative medications. The interactions and effects are specific to the type of substance used. For example, patients who inject heroin may have hardened veins, making it difficult to obtain IV access. Cocaine and amphetamines are central nervous system stimulants, which can increase blood pressure and precipitate cardiac arrest. Hallucinogens, or psychedelics, such as LSD and "shrooms" produce an altered state of consciousness and can interfere with perioperative medications, increasing the risk of hallucinations, anxiety, and paranoia.

Physical Assessment

Anatomy and Physiology

The nurse must have an understanding of basic anatomy and physiology concepts in order to conduct an accurate patient assessment. Each patient, at minimum, requires an assessment of the cardiac, respiratory, and renal systems prior to surgery. Knowledge of cardiac anatomy is necessary to auscultate heart sounds, including an apical pulse. **Electrocardiograms (ECGs)** are routinely performed preoperatively, and in order to accurately obtain an ECG, the nurse must correctly place the leads. Without a basic understanding of cardiac anatomy, the nurse can't perform this task.

Understanding anatomy of the respiratory system is essential in auscultating breath sounds accurately. If the nurse isn't sure where the right upper lobe of the lung is located, accurate assessment of breath sounds isn't possible.

In performing the renal assessment, the nurse should understand what lab values are associated with acute or chronic renal insufficiency. Also, if the nurse needs to perform a post-void bladder scan, they need to know which area of the lower pelvic region to place the ultrasound probe. If the patient is complaining of severe pain in the right flank area, the nurse should be aware that this could be related to a kidney issue.

Abnormal findings in any of these three categories warrant further investigation to ensure the patient is safe for surgery. The nurse's knowledge of anatomy and physiology enables the nurse to discern findings that deviate from the norm. Documentation of anatomical and physiological assessments provides a baseline for comparison postoperatively.

Nursing Process

The preoperative patient assessment includes obtaining subjective and objective data and is essential in formulating the patient's plan of care. Each step of the **nursing process** (assessment, diagnosis, planning, implementation, and evaluation) is used during the preoperative assessment.

During the initial step, the nurse performs subjective, objective, and psychosocial assessments. During the subjective assessment, the nurse allows the patient the opportunity to ask questions and evaluates the patient's knowledge of the procedure and what to expect during the process. The objective assessment is the data collection piece (lab values, vital signs, physical assessment, etc.). A psychosocial assessment addresses the patient's support systems, such as family, friends, and economic, as well as the patient's feelings. Common feelings patients have during this time are anxiety, fear, anger, hopelessness, worry, and feeling overwhelmed by their disease process. Sometimes the nurse can alleviate these feelings by explaining what to expect in the preoperative, intraoperative, and postoperative phases of care. The nurse should speak to the patient in terms the patient can easily understand. If the patient expresses a strong fear of death related to the surgery, the nurse should inform the surgeon. Because the patient's emotional state influences the body's stress response, the surgeon may choose to do the surgery at another time or cancel it altogether.

During the diagnosis phase, the nurse uses the assessment data and formulates nursing diagnoses.

The diagnoses guide the planning phase, where the nurse develops next steps in care. These steps involve nursing actions but may include steps to be taken by interdisciplinary team members. For example, if one diagnosis is knowledge deficit related to the surgical procedure, the nurse may ask the surgeon to review the plan with the patient and family again.

Once the nurse completes the planning process, implementation begins. Implementation often begins with educating the patient on the plans, expected outcomes, and how the patient can be involved in the plan of care. For example, if the nurse is implementing a postoperative pain management plan, the nurse should explain this to the patient during the preoperative phase, while the patient is (presumably) at their baseline. With the agreement of a negotiated pain level and the plan for postoperative pain medication and nonpharmacological pain management measures, the patient is more likely to achieve desired pain control.

The final phase of the nursing process is evaluation; however, evaluation happens across the continuum of the nursing process, not just at the end. The nurse frequently evaluates the effectiveness of care plans, adjusts as necessary, and reevaluates.

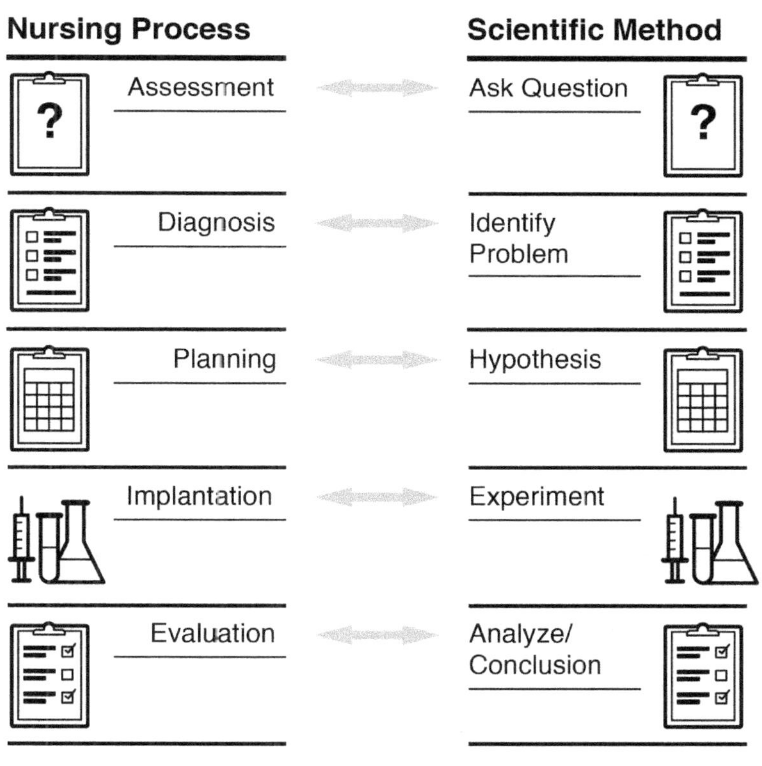

Focused Assessment

Prior to the surgical or invasive procedure, the nurse must perform a focused physical assessment. The focused assessment is dependent on the type of procedure being performed. However, an overview of the patient's health status will include an assessment of all major body systems.

For example, a patient undergoing abdominal surgery will require a focused gastrointestinal assessment. This may include inspecting the abdomen for distention, auscultating bowel sounds, and inquiring about the last meal and bowel movement. A focused integumentary assessment includes inspecting the skin for lesions, color, and hydration. Immobility during the perioperative period is a factor to consider for patients at risk for skin integrity issues. Respiratory assessments evaluate breath sounds, ease of breathing, and chest characteristics. A cardiovascular assessment will help determine the patient's ability to perfuse major organs. Assessments include inspection for jugular vein distention or edema and auscultation of heart sounds for rate and rhythm. Musculoskeletal assessments test muscle strength and ability to ambulate. Postoperative care includes early ambulation and mobility, so it is important for the nurse to assess a patient's range of motion and ability to perform activities of daily living.

A neurological assessment is imperative in the preoperative phase. A patient's level of consciousness, orientation, and speech pattern help determine their overall physical and mental state. Sensory and motor function should be documented and compared to postoperative findings. Intraoperative medications can alter a patient's coordination and response time. Any changes from the patient's baseline assessment should be promptly reported to the healthcare provider.

After a patient undergoes a procedure and is in the recovery phase, it is important to assess readiness for discharge from the post-anesthesia care unit (PACU). The nurse will use various tools to perform focused assessments. A commonly used instrument is the Aldrete scoring system. The Aldrete score ranges from 0 to 10, with 10 being the ideal score for discharge. The total score is determined by individual areas of assessment. The highest score for each assessment area is 2 points. Areas of assessment include consciousness, mobility, circulation, breathing, and color (oxygenation).

Pain Assessment

Pain is a subjective topic that varies by patient; therefore, healthcare professionals have a responsibility to combine clinical knowledge, personal expertise, and patient involvement in developing a safe and effective pain management plan. Unmanaged pain can lead to reduced quality of life, inability to complete basic tasks like eating, affect mood, and often leads to prolonged depression. In complex surgical cases, unmanaged pain can lead to poor recovery outcomes, including increased rates of infection and hormonal disruption. Pain management plans can employ a number of different techniques depending on the severity of the case.

Analgesia, Narcotics, NSAIDS, and Opioids

Analgesics is an umbrella term for a variety of pain-relieving pharmaceuticals that can include mild over-the-counter medications as well as prescription-strength medications that require close monitoring by a medical professional. Different categories of analgesics work by targeting different pathways to pain.

Nonsteroidal anti-inflammatory drugs (NSAIDS) include commonly recognized medications such as ibuprofen; prescription strength doses are simply much more concentrated than versions that can be bought over the counter. NSAIDS work by targeting areas of inflammation in the body that result in pain; consequently, they are most effective for pain situations involving muscles or soft tissues.

Opioids, a type of narcotic, are prescription-only medications that work by targeting nociceptors in the brain to reduce pathway signaling that result in the physical perception of pain. While these medications are often able to eliminate pain quickly, they can also cause extremely uncomfortable side effects, like severe nausea and dizziness, in some patients. Additionally, most narcotics are highly addictive, and an opioid epidemic is well-documented in the United States. These types of prescriptions should be carefully prescribed and monitored if they absolutely are required in patient treatment plans. As patients near the end of their prescription, they may need tailored treatment to avoid withdrawal symptoms.

Nonpharmacological Interventions

Non-pharmacological interventions can also manage pain. Depending on the cause and severity of pain, treatments like ice, heat, massage, breathing exercises, meditation, yoga, aromatherapy, hypnosis, and acupuncture can effectively eliminate or significantly reduce pain sensations.

Pain Assessment

Preoperative pain can be assessed in a number of ways, including visual and physical assessments, obtaining reports from the patient, and administering formal pain measurement scales. Visual and physical pain assessments may include noticing any conditions or injuries a patient has (for example, patients with a noticeable degree of kyphosis in their backs are expected to report a significant degree of muscular pain and tension along the spine) or noticing the intensity of pain that occurs with certain movements.

Patient self-reports of pain should be noted and taken seriously; however, patients who have previous prescriptions for narcotics or appear to desperately want them should be treated with extreme caution.

Finally, formal pain measurement instruments include numeric rating scales and verbal rating scales that patients work through with their healthcare providers to determine pain intensity. For preoperative patients, medical teams may choose a specific instrument with the patient prior to the procedure. During the preoperative period, medical teams may choose to review the instrument in detail with patients to ensure that they know how to properly report their pain levels. The selected instrument should then be utilized to continuously assess pain during the recovery period.

Anesthesia

During a procedure, patients may choose general anesthesia or localized anesthesia to mitigate potential pain. **General anesthesia** will place the patient into a fully sedated and unconscious state. This is most often used in major surgeries involving large muscle groups, organs, or other contexts that can be painful or otherwise cause patients the inability to remain still (as movement can cause critical surgical complications). Localized or **regional anesthesia** numbs sensation in a specific area but allows patients to remain alert and conscious. After surgical procedures are over, patients may experience a great deal of pain which can be managed through non-pharmacological mechanisms or prescription medications, including patient-controlled analgesia (PCA), where the patient controls a device that administers pain relief as needed.

Nursing Diagnoses

Nursing diagnoses are formulated after collecting assessment data, reviewing the medical record (including current medications), and interviewing the patient. Several **North American Nursing Diagnosis Administration (NANDA)** and Perioperative Nursing Data Set (PNDS) approved nursing diagnoses apply to the preoperative patient population. Common preoperative nursing diagnoses are anxiety regarding risks (including impaired skin integrity and mobility as well as death) and a lack of knowledge regarding the surgical procedure. Different age groups create an inherent risk for certain problems. Elderly patients are more at risk for impaired skin integrity, hypothermia, and dehydration. Using the nursing diagnoses, assessment findings, and collaboration with the interdisciplinary team, the plan of care is implemented to best meet the patient's needs. Evaluation of the plan of care occurs during the preoperative, perioperative, and postoperative phase, depending on the criteria being evaluated.

Advance Directives and DNR

Advance directives, such as a living will or durable power of attorney, are forms that state a patient's choices for treatment, including refusal of treatments, life support, and stopping treatments when the patient chooses. **Do not resuscitate (DNR)** status, and its varying types, is also included in advance directives. The preoperative interview should include discussion of advance directives and DNR status. If the patient has advance directives, a copy should be placed in the medical record, and they should be reviewed by the nurse and physician. If the patient has a code status of anything other than full resuscitation, a conversation among the surgeon, anesthesiologist, and patient is necessary to discuss the patient's wishes in detail. Older schools of thinking suggest all patients, regardless of preoperative DNR status, are considered full code while in the operating room; however, this is not true. A patient with DNR status of no intubation and no **cardiopulmonary resuscitation (CPR)** may proceed with the surgical procedure if the surgeon and anesthesiologist have a conversation with the patient and a plan is agreed upon among them.

Consent must be obtained by the patient if there is a change in status or a suspension of the DNR order during surgery. However, if the patient wishes to keep DNR status of no intubation and no CPR during surgery, the surgeon and/or anesthesiologist may deem the patient a nonsurgical candidate. If a patient is entering surgery with a DNR order of anything other than full code, this must be communicated to the entire surgical team and documented in the medical record.

Patient and Family Education

Patient and family education is a critical component of any operation. This allows patients and their families the opportunity to fully understand the procedure, voice questions or concerns, and empower them to play an active role in their health care. It can also foster rapport and a positive relationship between the patient party and the medical staff. Transparency, comprehensive education, and the sense of self-efficacy during medical procedures is often associated with better patient outcomes, increased patient satisfaction, and decreased complications during the recovery period.

Side Effects

Patients and their caretakers should be informed in detail of any potential side effects of an operation, including during the perioperative practices, associations with materials or medications used in the procedure, and effects that could occur during the recovery period. This allows patients to provide informed consent to the procedure, as well as manage their expectations and resources for the complete duration of their procedural timeline.

Resources for Patient/Family Education

One of the preoperative nurse's primary responsibilities is patient and family education. Regulatory bodies such as TJC and CMS clearly identify patient education as a need that must be fulfilled in order to promote optimal patient outcomes. The preoperative nurse is in a unique position of being able to provide education on the immediate next steps (entering the OR suite, monitoring, positioning, induction of anesthesia, emergence from anesthesia, transitioning to post-anesthesia care unit [PACU]) in addition to identifying discharge planning needs. Discharge planning begins at time of admission, and much education is based on preparing the patient and family on postoperative care at home.

Resources for education lie in a variety of areas. The nurse can verbalize the preoperative plan of care in addition to providing visual resources, such as written preoperative instructions. The nurse may provide a pamphlet or video for the patient and family. Hospital libraries and Internet databases are often good resources for educational materials. Some facilities offer preoperative classes, particularly with joint, spine, and cardiac surgical patients. Human resources such as case managers, disease-specific educators (i.e., diabetes educator, CHF educator), specialty physicians (endocrinologists, infectious disease physicians), social workers, chaplains, and physical therapists are beneficial to the nurse in providing specialized education to the patient and family.

It is important for the nurse to realize educational barriers and know how to address them. Anxiety is a common barrier to learning, and the patient and family may be overwhelmed by the entire process leading them to the preoperative area. The nurse may need to repeat the education several times for it to be "heard." Considering health literacy, the nurse must present the information in plain, clear language the patient and family can understand. If language barriers are present, the nurse can use an interpreter and material printed in the patient's language to ensure the proper delivery of information. During the educational process, the nurse should verify patient and family understanding of the information. This can be done by asking the patient and/or family to repeat back or paraphrase the information given to them.

Teach Back

The "Teach Back" method is an interactive educational technique that fosters rapport, communication, and information sharing between healthcare providers and patients. It encourages the healthcare providers to explain medical diagnoses, prognoses, and plans of care to patients in clear, non-medical terms. Then, patients are asked to explain the medical situation and plan of care to the healthcare professional, utilizing their own understanding. This empowers patients to actively engage in their care plans and understand their health in a new way. It also allows the healthcare provider to determine whether or not the patient has an appropriate understanding of their health situation and how to manage care once they are out of the medical setting. Providers should remain calm, compassionate, and responsive during this process, even if the patient is unable to correctly teach back right away.

Practice Quiz

1. An assessment of which physiological system is a minimum requirement during the preoperative assessment?
   a. Musculoskeletal
   b. Genitourinary
   c. Renal
   d. Central nervous

2. Knowledge of which aspect of the patient's respiratory anatomy would be MOST beneficial during the preoperative assessment?
   a. Location of right middle lobe
   b. Absence of right lower lobe
   c. Size of left upper lobe
   d. Breath sounds of left lower lobe

3. The preoperative nurse is assessing a patient scheduled for a left ventricular assist device (LVAD) insertion. Understanding the pathophysiology of congestive heart failure, which abnormality can the nurse expect to find during the preoperative assessment?
   a. Anuria
   b. Right facial drooping
   c. Absence of popliteal pulses
   d. 2+ bilateral lower extremity pitting edema

4. A newly diagnosed stage IV lung cancer patient is scheduled for insertion of an infusion port for long-term intravenous (IV) therapy. Based on this, which nursing intervention is MOST appropriate?
   a. Provide smoking cessation education to the patient.
   b. Allow time for the patient to express fears and provide emotional support.
   c. Ask the physician for a preoperative cardiology consult.
   d. Arrange for case management to set up cardiac rehab at discharge.

5. Which of the following describes the action created by a drug?
   a. Pharmacology
   b. Side effect
   c. Adverse reaction
   d. Intended effect

See answers on next page.

Answer Explanations

1. C: Each patient, at a minimum, requires an assessment of the cardiac, respiratory, and renal systems prior to surgery. Assessment of the musculoskeletal, genitourinary, and central nervous systems may be indicated, depending on the type of surgery scheduled or based on the patient's assessment findings. However, assessment of these systems is not a minimum requirement of all surgical patients.

2. B: Absence of the right lower lobe is important for the nurse to know because right lower lobe breath sounds will not be present in this patient. The general location of the right middle lobe is irrelevant, as is the size of the left upper lobe. The left lower lobe breath sounds may warrant further investigation of respiratory status, but only if they deviate from expected findings.

3. D: Pitting edema is an expected finding with CHF patients. Anuria, facial drooping, and absence of popliteal pulses are not part of the pathophysiology of CHF and are not expected findings in CHF patients.

4. B: The nurse should note that although the scheduled procedure may be minor, the patient's diagnosis may be quite serious. Understanding this, the nurse should allow more time for the patient to verbalize feelings and provide emotional support for the patient. Smoking cessation education, although important, is not the most important intervention at this time. Neither a cardiology consult nor cardiac rehab is indicated based on the information provided.

5. A: The nurse should review the pharmacology, or the action created by a drug, of the patient's current medications. Knowing the pharmacological effects of these medications and those of the scheduled preoperative medications can help keep the patient safe. Side effects and adverse reactions are included in the pharmacology. The intended effect does not include possible side effects or adverse reactions.

Individualized Plan of Care Development and Expected Outcome

Using the nursing process, a plan of care is created that reflects the goals, interventions, and expected outcomes set by the nurse. Steps involved in planning the care of the preoperative patient are modeled by evidence-based guidelines and surgical core measures.

- An individualized plan of care is developed considering the following criteria.
    - The nurse anticipates the physiological responses of the patient and formulates diagnoses that reflect identified risks and needs. Commonly identified risks in the preoperative patient are risk of infection, altered thermal response, and impaired skin integrity. Interventions related to these risks are incorporated in the plan of care.
    - Current Surgical Care Improvement Project (SCIP) measures are implemented by the surgical team preoperatively. These include preoperative antibiotic prophylaxis, administration of beta-blocker drugs in certain patients, and application of antiembolism stockings and/or compression devices.
    - The nurse prepares the patient for safety needs unique to preoperative patients. The patient may be exposed to radiation and laser during the procedure; measures are taken to minimize exposure to the patient and operative personnel. Fire safety measures include a fire extinguisher in the room and normal saline or sterile water on the sterile field if electrosurgery is used. Patient positioning is carefully examined, and the nurse ensures that proper anatomical alignment and padding are used.
    - The nurse identifies behavioral responses of the patient and family. Measures are taken to reduce anxiety and fear. Cultural and spiritual needs are met as appropriate. Comfort measures are used as much as possible. Pain management, including pain medication administration, may also be considered.
    - Age-specific needs are incorporated in the care plan as needed. This may include temperature regulation, alternate positioning methods, selecting smaller instruments (pediatric or neonatal patient), providing a tangible comfort item (blanket, toy), or consoling a crying or extremely fearful patient.
    - The nurse arranges for an interpreter to be present if a language barrier exists. If cultural or religious needs are identified, the nurse incorporates these into the plan whenever possible.
    - Ethical and legal guidelines are upheld according to professional standards. The nurse provides nonbiased, competent, safe care and practices within guidelines per institutional policies and procedures.
    - Interdisciplinary teams are used in providing evidence-based care. IDTs in the surgical setting can include radiology personnel, ultrasound technicians, pharmacists, laboratory staff, and consulting physicians.

- The nurse uses a patient-centered care model in practice. Patient-centered care dimensions include patient preferences, emotional support, physical comfort, information and education, continuity and transition, coordination of care, access to care, and family and friends. These aspects are considered on an individual basis. The nurse uses the patient-centered care model throughout the nursing process.

- Expected patient outcomes are identified by the nurse, and the plan of care is reflective of these. When deviations from the expected outcomes are identified, the nurse modifies the care plan and associated interventions.

- Standard precautions are adhered to by the nurse and the operative team to decrease the risk of hospital-acquired infection. Performing hand hygiene at the appropriate times is the number one measure health care professionals can take to minimize infection risk. PPE should be available at all times for the health care team's use.

Measurable Patient Outcomes

Ultimately, the purpose of education, care bundles, core measures, and guidelines is to promote the best possible **patient outcomes**. Patient outcomes are identified as high priority by nurses, physicians, patients, families, professional organizations, and governing bodies. One of the quality objectives of the **Affordable Care Act** (**ACA**), enacted in 2010, is fewer avoidable hospital readmissions. Avoidable hospital readmissions are considered negative outcomes for all parties involved, but especially for the patients. The **Institute for Healthcare Improvement (IHI)** is a worldwide driver of health care improvement and best patient outcomes. The IHI's work focuses on improvement capability, person- and family-centered care, patient safety, and quality, cost, and value. These focus groups are all aimed to improve patient outcomes.

The **Centers for Medicare and Medicaid Services (CMS)** was formed in 1977. CMS provides value-based incentives to providers and institutions by tying reimbursement to better patient outcomes. Conversely, CMS withholds reimbursement to institutions and providers if a patient is readmitted to the hospital within thirty days of discharge if the readmission is related to the same problem causing the initial hospitalization. For instance, a patient is admitted to the hospital with CHF exacerbation, treated, and released. Two weeks later, the patient is readmitted with CHF exacerbation. Neither the hospital nor the physician is reimbursed for care related to the readmission.

Another way of improving patient outcomes is with the use of **electronic health records** (**EHRs**). EHRs help health care providers to access complete and accurate health information in a timely fashion. EHRs have also been shown to reduce (and even prevent) medical errors due to misinterpretation of handwriting. EHRs also allow built-in systems designed to prevent treatment errors. TJC created the Surgical Care Improvement Project (SCIP) with the goal of substantially reducing negative patient outcomes (surgical mortality and morbidity), specifically **surgical site infection** (**SSI**) and venous thromboembolism (VTE). Nurses promote best patient outcomes by providing education to patients and families by utilizing best practice guidelines and using these in the nursing process.

Specific Interventions

Nurses must identify actual or potential problems that a perioperative patient may experience. The determination of a nursing diagnosis is influenced by the three stages of the perioperative experience (preoperative, intraoperative, and postoperative). A nursing diagnosis should have related risk factors and defining characteristics that serve as evidence of an actual or potential problem. Nursing interventions will be aimed at preventing or correcting existing problems.

For example, in the preoperative phase, the patient may be at risk for infection due to their medical history and physical assessment. Risk diagnoses typically do not have defining characteristics since the chosen diagnosis is a potential problem. A patient at risk for infection would have the following nursing diagnosis according to NANDA (an international organization responsible for standardizing terms used in diagnoses): risk for infection related to alteration in skin integrity, obesity, and history of smoking. The related factors would be specific to the patient's disease process. Nursing interventions would emphasize teaching about early mobilization, prepping the skin for surgery, and providing adequate hygiene and hydration.

During the intraoperative phase, the patient's condition can be altered by various processes, medications, and the procedure itself. The patient is usually sedated and immobile, increasing the risk of fluid volume depletion (or overload) and decreased cardiac output. Related factors include hemorrhage, administration of intravenous fluids, and secondary effects of anesthesia. Nursing interventions include continuous monitoring, patient positioning, and maintaining environmental safety.

Acute pain is a primary nursing diagnosis for a patient in the postoperative stage. The surgical procedure and intentional injury to the skin will result in physiological changes. The patient may experience an increase in blood pressure, pulse, and respirations. Facial grimacing and guarding behaviors are additional defining characteristics. Prompt recognition of signs and symptoms along with adequate pain management are key nursing interventions in the recovery period.

As with any other nursing process, an evaluation of the interventions must be performed to ensure that the outcomes were successfully met.

Specific Patient Considerations

Age-Specific Needs

In addition to understanding universally applicable needs, the preoperative nurse identifies age-specific needs in creating the patient's plan of care. Providing age-specific care requires knowledge of typical behaviors and processes within each developmental stage. Infants and children, adolescents, adults, and geriatric adults have different age-specific characteristics to integrate into planning nursing care. An infant's immune, renal, gastrointestinal, thermoregulatory, and pulmonary systems are not fully developed; therefore, infants are at increased risk of postoperative complications. The lack of an infant's circulating immunoglobulins increases the risk of infection. Conditions that affect electrolyte imbalance, such as diarrhea, dehydration, and NPO status, can cause fluid shifts and potentially acidosis.

Infants undergoing general anesthesia are prone to nausea and vomiting, and this can lead to deficient nutritional intake. Although all patients are at risk of hypothermia during surgery, infants are at particularly high risk due to their low body surface area and distribution of body fat. As compared to adults, children have a higher response to vasodilatation and vasoconstriction during exposure to heat and cold. The airways of infants and children are narrower than those of adults, and this increases the risk of airway obstruction. Children and infants alike have increased oxygen consumption demands and are less tolerant of hypoxia. The pain response systems of infants are not yet fully developed. Because of this, nurses use pain scales based on facial expressions, body movements, crying, and the ability of caregivers to console the infants in pain assessments. Children, like infants, are at increased risk for hypothermia and gastrointestinal complications.

Although older children (between five and eighteen years of age) are generally able to verbally express pain level, they tend to have a lower pain tolerance than adults. Patients from infancy to age two often experience separation anxiety. School-aged children are concrete thinkers, so the health care team should use concrete communication rather than vague statements left to interpretation. Adolescents have unique emotional and psychosocial needs. An adolescent's sense of identity and desire for autonomy drives the nurse to include this patient in communication related to surgery. The heightened importance of body image creates anxiety around postoperative scars and disfigurement related to surgery. The nurse may identify decisional conflict and situational low self-esteem as nursing diagnoses in this age group.

Adults are the lowest-risk age group from a physiological standpoint. Knowledge deficit related to the disease process or surgical course of treatment is a common nursing diagnosis in adult patients. Adults often seek to understand their disease process, treatment options, and how to best comply with the postoperative treatment plan. Adults are also the primary family caregivers, and an adult may struggle with anxiety and fear related to loss of control and ability to care for children or aging parents while recovering from surgery. Financial concerns related to time away from work can contribute to anxiety related to the surgical process.

Older adults have decreased physiological reserves and are less able to bounce back from surgery. Like infants and children, an aging adult's immune, thermoregulatory, pulmonary, and renal systems are less functional. Aging adults often take multiple medications; the side effects of multiple medications contribute to a phenomenon called **polypharmacy**. This increases the likelihood of experiencing medication-to-medication reactions. Some surgeries represent a loss of body function to aging adult patients, and they often worry about becoming a burden to their families. Additionally, this age group is at higher risk of falling due to impaired neurological function and mobility.

Behavioral Responses

Not only does the surgical process have physiological effects on the body, but it also induces **behavioral responses**. Behavioral responses to surgery include, but are not limited to, the following: anxiety, fear, agitation, depression, noncompliance, altered body image, stress, and disturbances in eating and sleep patterns. Pediatric patients may display separation anxiety, fear, and loss of trust in the parents and health care team. The fear of dying is one of the most common causes of preoperative anxiety. Patients often verbalize being afraid of not waking up from surgery. Anticipating postoperative pain and not knowing if it will be controlled adequately can certainly promote anxiety and fear. This is one reason the nurse performs a preoperative pain assessment and education on the postoperative plan for pain management. Allowing the nurse and patient to negotiate a tolerable pain level together gives the patient a sense of ownership and control in the care plan, helping to decrease anxiety and fear.

A patient may also experience postoperative anxiety and fear awaiting biopsy results, as this can be life changing for the patient and their family. The patient may feel a loss of control overall, and this contributes to agitation, noncompliance with treatments set forth by someone other than himself/herself, and sometimes anger with the health care team or with everyone in general. Depression may be a behavioral response. For instance, a cardiac transplant recipient often suffers from depression as a result of internalizing the fact that the transplant was able to take place because a person lost their life. The patient may feel undeserving of the gift that has been received: a second chance at life. For this reason, a cardiac transplant workup consists of a psychiatric evaluation. Some patients respond to the stress of the surgical process with eating and sleeping disturbances. Recognizing the patient's individual behavioral responses and incorporating these responses into the plan of care helps provide holistic patient care.

Community Resources

After a patient undergoes a surgical procedure, the care that follows focuses on recovery and rehabilitation. The type of discharge resources needed will be dependent on the patient's surgical experience. The nurse will need to collaborate with the interdisciplinary team, such as case managers and social workers, to provide the patient with the necessary community resources to achieve an optimal health status. For example, a patient with a total hip replacement will require physical therapy during the recovery process to ensure full mobility is restored. Depending on the patient's age, additional caregiver services may be required for assistance with activities of daily living.

Cultural/Ethnic Influences

A patient's perception of the surgical experience will be influenced by their cultural and ethnic background. It is important for the nurse to assess the patient's sociocultural needs during the preoperative period. The patient's background may require individualized nursing interventions to meet their needs. Some of those needs may include food preferences, translation services, and rituals performed pre- and post-surgery. For example, in the Chinese culture, yin (cold) and yang (hot) foods provide balance. In the immediate postoperative period, the patient may request specific foods to aid in recovery. Additionally, the nurse must always be prepared to request interpreter services for patients with a language barrier.

Disease Processes

Individualized care plans for perioperative patients should focus on existing disease processes, as applicable. A medical history will help determine what actual or potential problems the nurse should address throughout the surgical experience. For example, a patient with history of diabetes mellitus is identified as having a risk for infection or delayed wound healing after surgery due to altered glycemic control. The nurse would establish interventions that aim to control the patient's serum glucose. Additionally, patient education regarding postoperative care and glucose control are imperative. In the intraoperative period, careful monitoring for hypo or hyperglycemia can prevent adverse events.

Diversity

When reviewing a patient's care plan, nurses must take into consideration the diversity of personal values. Subcultures are influenced by various factors such as occupation, family make-up, and social norms. Although a patient may identify as a particular race or ethnicity, the nurse must be careful not to assume certain practices or beliefs typically associated with the culture. For example, in Eastern medicine, an imbalance in nature is believed to cause illness and disease. Although this may be a common belief amongst people from certain regions, a patient may be accustomed to different health practices and beliefs based on their upbringing and lifestyle.

Family Patterns

Family dynamics must be assessed to ensure successful recovery of the operative patient. During the preoperative phase, the nurse should assess the structure of the patient's family. Family patterns are diverse and can include two or more people that are related or unrelated to each other. Patients may consider significant others, friends, co-workers, or other members of the community to be part of their family. Not all family patterns are traditional, and it is important for nurses to determine the patient's capability to complete plan of care tasks successfully, whether individually or with family support.

Institutional Resources

Institutional resources should be taken into consideration when creating, reviewing, and evaluating a perioperative patient's plan of care. The resources available are dependent on the type of facility and staff capability. A plan of care cannot be successfully implemented without the necessary resources within the institution. For example, a patient with an ankle surgery requires physical therapy for a successful recovery. However, an outpatient surgical center may not employ physical therapists, and the patient will not be admitted to an inpatient unit. Although mobility would still be a crucial consideration in the patient's care plan, the immediate interventions and timeline for outcome completion may need to be revised.

Legal and Ethical Standards

Patients have a legal right to be informed of their plan of care. When developing outcomes and interventions, the nurse and healthcare providers must discuss the care plan with the patient. The patient has a right to agree or disagree with the proposed plan of care. Nurses must also be cognizant of the patient's ability to provide informed consent for an invasive procedure. The nurse may need to refer the plan of care to the next of kin or to the patient's medical power of attorney. In all cases, the nurse must remain an advocate for the patient's and implement a plan of care that acts in the patient's best interest.

Patient Rights and Responsibilities

A patient who provides consent to treatment maintains legal privileges—known as patient rights—regarding their care. The plan of care that is developed for the perioperative patient includes pre, intra, and postoperative interventions. The nurse is held accountable for protecting the rights of patients while the plan of care is developed at every stage of the surgical experience. After the plan of care is discussed with the patient, they have the right to accept, request a revision, or decline the plan. The nurse must work collaboratively with the patient and the interdisciplinary team to ensure all parties are in agreement with the care being provided and the expectations of the patient's involvement in their care.

Perioperative Safety

All plans of care should emphasize patient safety. Perioperative safety is a priority for achieving successful patient outcomes. Expected patient outcomes and nursing interventions should be developed according to the patient's priority needs. For example, an older adult patient undergoing a hip replacement will have multiple safety needs throughout the surgical experience. In the pre and intraoperative phases, the nurse must ensure that the patient is vitally stable to undergo the procedure, taking into consideration the patient's age and reaction to medications intraoperatively. Postoperatively, the nurse must consider the patient's ability to ambulate on their own, their risk of falls, and injury prevention during the rehabilitation period.

Physiologic Response

Physiological response refers to surgery-specific reactions produced by individuals who undergo a medical procedure or related trauma. This response appears to take the same course across most individuals and includes temporary nervous, endocrine, and metabolic system changes. Immediately upon a traumatic event (such as surgery), the body produces stress hormones (such as cortisol, adrenaline, and catecholamines), excess growth hormones, and excess insulin. This creates systemic inflammation in the body. In the ensuing days, the body's metabolic system shows an ebb-and-flow effect through cyclic decreases and increases in cardiac output, oxygenation, and glucose consumption until the body is able to return to a state of homeostasis. Post-surgery, homeostasis is supported through medical interventions of nutritional supplementation (especially of glucose and amino acids), electrolyte rebalancing, and pharmaceuticals to decrease the metabolic stress on the body.

Spirituality

The surgical experience can be a challenging time for patients. Although many surgeries are elective, others are medically necessary and can often result in loss of a limb, functionality, or altered cognitive function. When developing a plan of care for a patient, the nurse must assess the patient's spirituality. A patient's faith and religious practices will influence how they perceive their health and well-being. Nursing interventions for the established care plan should be mindful of the patient's spiritual beliefs while also considering their physical well-being. For example, a patient may request frequent periods of privacy to perform a religious prayer. However, during the postoperative period, the nurse may need to assess the patient's vital signs frequently. Planning a timing strategy to achieve both outcomes would be the ideal goal.

Evaluating Patient Responses to Plan of Care

Successful evaluation of the plan of care is determined by the completion of patient outcomes. Care plans differ at every stage of the perioperative experience. The expected outcomes are based on the patient's ability to reach the goals and the nurse's ability to implement all interventions.

In the preoperative phase, a common goal for patients is an understanding of the procedure and subsequent recovery expectations. A patient is deemed prepared for surgery when they are able to consent to the procedure, understand the risk and benefits, verbalize the expected outcomes, and demonstrate the ability to perform postoperative activities. When a goal is not achieved, the nurse must ensure that any deficiencies in patient knowledge are addressed prior to advancing to the intraoperative phase.

Intraoperative outcomes are dependent on the patient's health status during the procedure. The nurse must prioritize expected outcomes based on the patient's responses to anesthesia, medications, and the procedure. For example, common intraoperative outcomes include maintaining fluid and electrolyte balance, remaining free of accidental injury from surgical instruments, and maintaining normothermia. Evaluation of the outcomes would be based on the patient's cardiovascular status, safety, and vital sign stability.

Postoperative evaluation of goals and expected outcomes can be short or long-term. A patient in the recovery phase of a procedure can achieve an expected outcome immediately, or it may take days, weeks, months, or even longer to observe results. Many facilities have nurse advice lines that follow up with patients postoperatively to ensure they are meeting their expected outcomes. For example, a patient undergoing cataract surgery may demonstrate an immediate improvement in vision after the procedure. The patient's goal of improved sensory perception can be evaluated immediately after treatment. However, a patient who has a repair of a lower extremity fracture will require several weeks of rehabilitation before the goal of intact mobility can be evaluated.

Updating Plan of Care

The outcomes set during the planning phase of the nursing process often require revisions. The revisions are based on the patient's inability to meet the stated goals, or the patient's change in health status. The patient also has the right to request revisions to the plan of care, and the nurse should work to ensure that the goals are patient-centered and realistic for each situation.

Updates to the plan of care can occur during the implementation or evaluation phase of the nursing process. When performing interventions, the nurse can determine if the patient can realistically perform the activities stated in the plan of care. The plan of care can be modified, or an attempt can be made to encourage the patient to meet the outcomes. The determination of a goal being met, not met, or partially met is achieved when the patient performs the interventions outlined in the plan of care. The nurse can then modify the care plan, if needed, to ensure that the outcomes align with the patient's current health status.

Modifications to the plan of care should be communicated to the patient, and education regarding the new expected outcomes should be provided. Revisions can include a change in nursing diagnosis, stating a more realistic outcome, adjusting the time criteria of goals, or changing the nursing interventions. The patient should be informed of the reason why the plan of care needs to be revised and how they will benefit from the modifications.

For example, an initial outcome for a patient undergoing abdominal surgery may be to tolerate fluids within the first 24 hours postoperatively. After the nurse provides a liquid diet, the patient becomes nauseous and vomits. The goal has not been met. At this point, the nurse would consider revising the time criteria or incorporating alternative interventions to help the patient achieve the expected outcome.

Critical Thinking Skills

The perioperative experience can result in multiple patient complications. Invasive procedures carry risks ranging from infection, hemorrhage, accidental injury, hemodynamic instability, and prolonged recovery periods. At every stage, the nurse must use critical thinking skills to maintain the patient's health and safety. Critical thinking skills are acquired through years of bedside experience and knowledge gained from training programs and continuing education. Nurses must use a variety of problem solving and intuitive skills to ensure patient care issues are prevented or addressed in a timely manner.

In the preoperative stage, nurses must use critical thinking skills to determine if a patient is stable enough to undergo an invasive procedure. Although the determination is made collaboratively with other members of the healthcare team, nurses oversee the entire patient experience. It is crucial to perform interventions such as conducting a physical assessment, reviewing laboratory results, and assessing a patient's physical and mental well-being before the procedure. Any concerns must immediately be reported to the healthcare provider. For example, if a patient will be sedated for a prolonged period of time, a respiratory assessment is a priority. Should the nurse auscultate crackles in the lungs or note any respiratory abnormality, the patient may need further screening to determine the stability of their health status. Anticipating potential problems and promptly reporting abnormal results is an essential critical thinking skill that can prevent intraoperative complications.

During the intraoperative stage, patient safety begins with performing a time-out procedure. This protocol ensures verification of the correct patient, operative site, and procedure. Throughout the procedure, the patient is at risk for developing complications such as hypothermia, infection, and electrolyte imbalances. The circulating nurse must carefully observe operating room practices to ensure the patient's health is maintained. For example, if a surgeon breaks sterile technique, the nurse anticipates a risk for infection and has the responsibility to voice the concern and facilitate new supplies.

Postoperatively, the nurse must assess the patient's ability to recover. Interventions in the immediate postoperative period include monitoring vital signs, maintaining fluids, controlling pain, and assessing the surgical site. Any abnormalities that can hinder recovery should be reported immediately. For example, if the nurse notices decreased capillary refill and discoloration to an extremity that underwent a wound debridement, these findings may indicate a potential problem with wound healing and recovery. Before the nurse receives orders from the healthcare provider, interventions to maintain circulation would be implemented (i.e., maintaining a stable blood pressure, ensuring adequate hydration, and preventing immobility).

Practice Quiz

1. Sympathetic and parasympathetic responses are components of which physiological system?
   a. Central nervous system
   b. Hepatic system
   c. Immunological system
   d. Cardiovascular system

2. From a cardiovascular standpoint, which piece of data provides the nurse with the best insight as to how the patient will tolerate activity postoperatively?
   a. The patient's incentive spirometry volume is 500 mL.
   b. No history of type 2 diabetes is noted.
   c. The patient denies shortness of breath in activities of daily living.
   d. Lab values show a serum creatinine level of 0.8.

3. Which of the following is a behavioral response to surgery?
   a. Increased heart rate
   b. Increased oxygen consumption
   c. Decreased clearance of respiratory secretions
   d. Sleep pattern disturbance

4. In recognizing age-specific needs, the nurse identifies which group to be at highest risk of hypothermia during surgery?
   a. School-aged children
   b. Infants
   c. Adolescents
   d. Aging adults

5. Ethnicity, ancestry, religion, and culture domains are encompassed in which nursing theory?
   a. Nightingale's Environment Theory
   b. Leininger's Transcultural Nursing Theory
   c. Erikson's Modeling and Role Modeling Theory
   d. Kolcaba's Theory of Comfort

See answers on next page.

Answer Explanations

1. A: The central nervous system (CNS) is composed of two domains: sympathetic and parasympathetic. The hepatic system involves the liver and portal veins. Neither the immunological nor cardiovascular systems are specific to sympathetic and parasympathetic domains.

2. C: Determining the patient's functional capacity is a good indicator of surgical risk, and this is an indicator of cardiovascular well-being. Incentive spirometry volume addresses pulmonary health. Type 2 diabetes is related to endocrine functioning. Serum creatinine levels are indicative of renal function.

3. D: Behavioral responses to surgery include, but are not limited to: anxiety, fear, agitation, depression, noncompliance, altered body image, stress, and disturbances in eating and sleep patterns. Increased heart rate, increased oxygen consumption, and decreased clearance of respiratory secretions are all physiological responses.

4. B: Although all patients are at risk of hypothermia during surgery, infants are at particularly high risk due to their low body surface area and distribution of body fat. All patients undergoing surgery (including school-aged children, adolescents, and aging adults) are at risk of hypothermia related to the surgical process, but infants are at the highest risk.

5. B: Madeleine Leininger was the first nurse to emphasize cultural care. According to Leininger, cultural care is achieved through "cognitively based assistive, supportive, facilitative, or enabling acts or decisions that are mostly tailor-made to fit with individual group's or institution's cultural values, beliefs, and lifeways." Transcultural Nursing Theory encompasses the domains of ethnicity, ancestry, religion, and culture. Nightingale's Environment Theory relates to nursing as a calling, art, and science. Erikson's Modeling and Role Modeling Theory speaks to respect for the patient's uniqueness. Kolcaba's Theory of Comfort prioritizes comfort in the forefront of health care.

Intraoperative Activities

Patient Care and Safety

Using the nursing process, a plan of care is created that reflects the goals, interventions, and expected outcomes set by the nurse. Steps involved in planning the care of the intraoperative patient are modeled by evidence-based guidelines and surgical core measures.

- The perioperative nurse optimizes physiological responses of the patient in the following ways.
  - Body temperature is maintained by the use of warming blankets and warm intravenous fluids in order to prevent hypothermia.
  - Surgical care improvement project (SCIP) measures, such as antibiotic prophylaxis and hair removal, are implemented by the surgical team to reduce the risk of SSI.
  - Tissue perfusion is assessed by monitoring the patient's skin color, temperature, and blood pressure.
- Patient and personnel safety are monitored and maintained.
  - Hazardous chemicals are handled according to precautionary measures listed on product labels.
  - Fire safety precautions are taken, as indicated by the type of surgical case. These precautions include ensuring the availability of a fire extinguisher, ensuring the availability of sterile saline or water on the surgical field for any case using laser or electrosurgical cautery, and following laser safety guidelines according to the type of laser used.
  - Smoke plumes are minimized by using smoke evacuators.
  - Radiation exposure to the perioperative team and the patient is minimized by the use of lead aprons, glasses, and drapes.
  - The surgeon, anesthesiologist, and perioperative nurse are active in the patient positioning process, promoting safety practices for safe patient positioning. Padding, proper anatomical alignment, and limb support are ensured.
- Patient care is optimized based on behavioral responses including patient comfort, anxiety management, and pain management. Pharmacological and nonpharmacological methods are used to promote patient comfort. The perioperative nurse also considers cultural, spiritual, and ethical issues when implementing nursing interventions.
- The surgical site is prepared according to best practice guidelines in preventing SSI. Examples include hair removal with clippers when hair is present at the incisional area and use of skin prep solution according to manufacturer instructions.

- Procedure-specific protective materials are utilized according to potential hazard risk. These include lead aprons, eye goggles, and drapes for radiology exposure, and laser goggles for laser cases.
- The perioperative nurse monitors the effects of pharmacological and anesthetic interventions to ensure the desired outcome is achieved. For example, the patient's pain level is reevaluated after administration of pain medication.
- The perioperative nurse assists in anesthesia management by monitoring vital signs, assisting with anesthesia induction, positioning the patient along with the anesthesiologist and surgeon, and assisting with airway management.
- Environmental factors are monitored in the following ways.
    - The operating room temperature is maintained according to healthcare facility policy. Generally, this is between sixty-eight and seventy-five degrees Fahrenheit.
    - The perioperative nurse ensures proper air exchange, room traffic pattern, humidity, and sterile field are maintained.
- Aseptic technique is followed by maintaining a sterile field.
    - The perioperative nurse ensures adherence to sterile technique by the surgical team.
    - Breaks in technique are resolved, if possible. In the case of gross contamination, the perioperative nurse ensures proper wound class documentation and implementation of measures to reduce risk of SSI.
- The sterility of surgical equipment is ensured by checking expiration dates, sterilization indicators, and integrity of packaging of instruments and supplies.
- Surgical equipment is tested and used according to manufacturer IFU. Manufacturer IFU documents are readily available for reference.
- Patient privacy and modesty are provided by covering the patient with a gown and/or blankets, when possible. The perioperative nurse uncovers the patient (as indicated) after sedation or anesthesia induction.
- The perioperative nurse verifies the name and type of all surgical specimens with the surgeon.
- The perioperative nurse ensures specimens are labeled correctly and accurately, according to healthcare facility policy. This typically includes patient name, date of birth, specimen type, and initials of person verifying the specimen.
- Prior to opening a surgical implant to the sterile field, the perioperative nurse verifies the type of implant, size (if applicable), and expiration date. The perioperative nurse verifies preparation requirements for the implant, such as a normal saline rinse. Documentation of surgical implant is entered into the medical record, and implant record is kept in the surgical department.

- Surgical explants are recorded into the patient's medical record and in the surgical department. The explanted item is routed to pathology department or disposed of according to healthcare facility policy.
- Containers for medications and solutions on the surgical field are labeled with type of medication or solution, along with concentration.
- Surgical counts are performed according to best practice guidelines. Counts are performed prior to skin incision, at the beginning of closure of body cavity or first skin layer, and during closure of final skin layer.
- Universal Protocol is followed:
    - Verification of surgical site is performed prior to patient entry into operating room.
    - Site marking is performed for any procedure involving the left or right side of the body, or left or right organ (i.e., kidney, lung).
    - Surgical time out is performed according to WHO checklist.
- The perioperative nurse maintains accurate and complete documentation of nursing care during the intraoperative period. Key elements included in perioperative nursing documentation are surgical counts, skin prep, positioning, implementation of nursing diagnoses and outcomes, and level of consciousness at time of transfer to next level of care.
- The perioperative nurse and anesthesia provider manage the hemodynamic needs of the patient. These include administration of intravenous fluids and blood or blood products.
- Ergonomics and proper body mechanics are utilized during patient care. The perioperative nurse utilizes safe patient mobilization equipment during patient transfer from stretcher to operating room bed, and during patient positioning.

Safe Practices

Patient and Personnel Safety

Patient and personnel safety are both paramount in perioperative nursing. Keeping the patient safe is arguably the most important aspect of patient care. **Patient safety** is influenced by multiple factors in concert with each other. The **Institute of Medicine (IOM)** released a report in 1999 titled *To Err Is Human: Building a Safer Health System*. This report brought attention to the issue of patient safety. As a result of the report, the IOM instituted six recommendations for improvement of patient safety. The recommendations are as follows: healthcare that is safe, effective, patient-centered, timely, efficient, and equitable. Addressing these objectives requires action from all parties involved in patient care, from patients to hospital administrators.

The Joint Commission (TJC) is an organization founded in 1951 with the mission of continuously improving healthcare for the public. TJC evaluates healthcare organizations and accredits them based on safe and effective care standards. Universal Protocol was developed by TJC in 2004 as an effort to prevent wrong site, wrong procedure, and wrong person surgery.

The **World Health Organization (WHO)** developed a surgical safety checklist, and the use of this checklist is considered a standard of care. The checklist highlights steps to be taken to ensure patient safety in the perioperative realm. An organizational culture of safety develops over time and takes commitment from all members of the organization. Safety is everyone's responsibility.

The Institute for Healthcare Improvement's (IHI) focus on patient safety includes integration of safety across the continuum of care and developing new tools for institutional leadership to address safety concerns. Human factors that affect patient safety are knowledge, skill, and attitude. Knowledge is acquired on a continuous basis, because evidence-based practice is constantly evolving. The skillset of the perioperative team members should be validated with evidence-based care guidelines. Attitudes of the perioperative team should be patient-centered and reflect safety as a top priority.

Measures to ensure **personnel safety** in the perioperative environment should be considered in the establishment of practice guidelines and protocols. The **Occupational Safety and Health Administration (OSHA)**, a part of the United States Department of Labor, was created in 1970. Its mission is to assure safe and healthful working conditions. Under OSHA laws and guidelines, employers are required to provide a safe work environment.

Personnel safety concerns in the perioperative environment include distractions and noise, staffing, safe patient mobilization, bullying and violence, chemical and drug hazards, biohazards, and sharps safety. Measures to minimize distractions and noise in the perioperative environment should be implemented as part of a culture of safety. An example of this is establishing a no-distraction zone in medication preparation areas. Noise in the operating room should be kept to a minimum, with side conversations being kept to a minimum.

Safe staffing ratios are essential for the perioperative team members to function in a safe, effective manner. Nurses working in short-staffing conditions are prone to fatigue and are more likely to make errors and endure injuries. The availability and use of safe patient mobilization devices are ways to improve personnel safety. Education on the use of these devices should be revisited periodically and documented in the personnel file. The act of bullying is defined as repeated, unwanted, harmful actions that are meant to threaten, humiliate, sabotage, or intimidate someone. According to the American Nurses Association (ANA), bullying in nursing is prevalent in all settings. Workplace violence includes physical and verbal abuse endured in the workplace. Both workplace bullying and violence negatively impact personnel safety. A culture of zero tolerance of bullying and workplace violence is imperative to personnel safety.

Nurses are at risk for chemical and biohazard exposure in the perioperative environment. Personnel should refer to the institution's hazardous materials (HAZMAT) manual for specific information about chemicals and biohazards used in the perioperative environment. This information should be presented to personnel at the beginning of employment. Potential sharps hazards in the perioperative setting should be identified, and action plans should be set to reduce exposure to them. Safety sharps devices should be used whenever possible to minimize the risk of injury for sharps. Intravenous catheter introducers and surgical knife handles are available with built-in safety devices to cover the sharp in a hands-free manner before and after use.

Surgical Care Improvement Project (SCIP)

The **Surgical Care Improvement Project (SCIP)** took place between 2005 and 2010. It was a quality-driven, nation-wide initiative aimed at reducing surgical complications and improving patient outcomes by establishing standardized guidelines for perioperative, operative, and postoperative patient care. These guidelines included directives such as strictly timed antibiotic administration, glucose monitoring, stringent patient preparation requirements, and practices to minimize the risk of postoperative infections. The project produced best practices and core measures that were compiled into a specifications manual; this serves as a benchmarking tool used by The Joint Commission to ensure sustained quality in the surgical setting.

Chemical

Chemical exposure refers to contact with or exposure to a chemical substance by touching, inhaling, or consuming it. Poisoning, which is one type of chemical exposure, is defined as the ingestion of, inhalation of, or skin contact with a substance that impairs health or kills a living organism.

There are treatments available only for certain types of poisons, and the possibility of an individual recovering from an accidental or intentional ingestion or inhalation of a harmful, poisonous agent is fundamentally determined by the amount of the agent absorbed by the body and how swiftly treatment to reverse the toxic effects of the poison is initiated. Some poisons can be detrimental to the lungs if inhaled and injurious to the esophagus and stomach lining if swallowed. Central nervous system (CNS) impairment can occur from alcohol poisoning or overdosing on prescription pain medications or antidepressants.

Young children are at an increased risk of accidental poisoning, as they are naturally inquisitive and curious about the world around them. To help prevent poisoning in children, all lower and upper cabinets in the home, especially in the kitchen and bathrooms, should be locked and bottles should be childproofed. The visual attractiveness of some cleaning products today makes it such that they are particularly alluring for children. For this reason, such products (e.g., Tide Pods, Fabuloso) should be kept out of reach of very young children. The elderly are also at a heightened probability of poisoning due to diminished eyesight and impaired memory. Under these circumstances, all medications should be locked away from the elderly person and only administered by a medical professional or a family member who has been educated about the dosage, route, reason for the medication, common side effects, and drug interactions and contraindications.

Some agents that are used for everyday gardening and farming, like pesticides, can be harmful to the eyes and skin if an individual does not take the proper protective precautions. There are three levels of pesticide poisoning: mild, moderate, and severe

Signs and symptoms of mild pesticide poisoning include, but are not limited to, mucous membrane, throat, and skin irritation; headache; dizziness; thirst; nausea; diarrhea; sweating; weakness or fatigue; and changes in mood. Moderate pesticide poisoning symptoms include excessive salivation, vomiting, abdominal cramps, difficulty swallowing or breathing, diaphoresis, trembling, inability to control muscular movements, and mental confusion. Severe pesticide poisoning signs include inability to breathe, chemical burns on the skin, loss of reflexes, unconsciousness, and death. In this type of poisoning, the CNS is severely affected.

Organophosphates are a type of synthetic insecticide known to be harmful to mammals, including humans. They are commonly used in agriculture. Acute symptoms of harmful exposure include headache, gastrointestinal effects, and malaise, while long-term exposure may be linked to nervous system issues, neurotransmitter disruption, and cancers such as leukemia and lymphoma. Some preliminary studies indicate that exposure may also cause reproductive and developmental harm. The

United States has banned many (though not all) organophosphates, but they are still used to manage agriculture in several other countries from which the United States imports food.

When caring for a patient who has ingested, inhaled, or been exposed to any harmful or poisonous substance, a nurse must know what was absorbed, how it was absorbed, and how much was absorbed. Knowing this information will allow a nurse to determine the best course of medical treatment. Basic therapies for the management of acute poisoning and exposure include washing the affected area (skin, eyes) with soap and water and inducing vomiting, but these are only applicable and effective with certain types of contaminants. If a corrosive cleaning agent (e.g., bleach, sodium hydroxide) is swallowed, vomiting is not the best way to rid the system of it. Anything caustic that is ingested burns the throat, esophagus, and small intestine as it makes its descent downward into the stomach, so it stands to reason that if that same product is forcibly removed from the digestive system through vomiting, it will also burn coming back up.

Gastric lavage is usually indicated when the patient has ingested a possibly life-threatening amount of a harmful substance and presents to the emergency department within one hour of intake. It involves flushing the stomach with saline in an attempt to remove the poison. Activated charcoal is sometimes given and has been proven to reduce the amount of poison absorbed if administered within one hour of ingestion.

Electrical

An electrical injury (electrocution) is defined as an instance in which an electrical current passes through a living organism. This type of injury occurs when electrical equipment is not stored properly, maintained in good working order, or grounded. Before operating any electrical equipment, an individual should inspect all electrical cords and outlets for uncovered, fraying, or damaged wires. One should never operate any unfamiliar electrical equipment or any electrical equipment near water or a water source.

There are different types of electrical burns: direct contact, electrical arcs, flame, and flash. With a direct contact burn, the current will pass straight through the body and cause damage to both the surface of the skin and deeper tissues. Electrical arc burns result when current sparks are formed between objects and cause deep thermal burns when they come into contact with the skin. A flame burn occurs when clothing ignites and burns the skin. A flash burn is the result of heat from a nearby electrical arc causing a thermal burn but not entering the body. Electrical injuries can result in temporary or prolonged unconsciousness, cardiac or respiratory arrest, renal failure, permanent brain damage, and, in some instances, death.

A patient presenting to the emergency department after an electrical injury may be unconscious, have suffered some sort of arrest, and/or have severe burns. A nurse must perform a thorough assessment to determine the type of burn and full extent of the injuries. Lab studies to perform include, but are not limited to, complete blood count (CBC), electrolyte panel, creatinine, and arterial blood gases (ABGs). Imaging studies to be considered include head computed tomography (CT) (especially if the patient was thrown from the electrical source), chest radiography, and cervical/spine imaging. An ECG will usually be done on any adult who has suffered an electrical injury, especially if that patient suffered a loss of consciousness, chest pain, arrhythmia, or myocardial infarction (heart attack).

Immediate nursing care will focus on maintaining a patent airway, monitoring circulation and establishing intravenous (IV) access, cervical spine immobilization, wound care, and, in extreme electrical burn instances, surgical consultation. If the electrical burn is very severe, the patient may be transferred to a burn and trauma center for more specialized treatment and therapy.

Complications that may arise after an electrical injury mainly depend on whether the injury was low voltage (less than 1000 volts) or high voltage (1000 volts or greater). With a low-voltage injury, recovery centers around the occurrence and interval of unconsciousness. The longer the patient was unconscious, the worse the prognosis. Any patient unconscious for 24 hours or greater has a slim chance of a full recovery. With low-voltage injuries, disfigurement can be minimized, but scarring is almost a certainty. In the event of a high-voltage injury, a patient can survive with massive burns, but potential amputation remains a concern, and traumatic injury significantly increases the rate of mortality.

Fire

RACE is an acronym used for fire safety purposes. It stands for Rescue, Alarm, Contain, Extinguish. It advises users to "RACE to safety" by removing themselves and others from dangerous fire situations; activating available fire alarms and alerting emergency services; containing the area housing the fire by closing windows, doors, and other entry points; and attempting to extinguish the fire if it does not pose a direct threat to the user. PASS is an acronym used when employing a fire extinguishing device. It stands for Pull, Aim, Squeeze, Sweep. Users should pull the pin that allows the extinguisher to work, aim at the base of the fire, squeeze the lever that controls the flow of the extinguishing substance, and sweep the device in long strokes across the flames until the fire is extinguished or emergency services have arrived.

Hazardous Waste Management

According to the Institute of Hazardous Materials Management (IHMM), a **hazardous material** is defined as "any item that has the potential to cause harm to humans, animals, or the environment, either by itself or through interaction with other factors." A hazardous item may be biological, chemical, radiological, and/or physical in nature. Agencies such as the United States Environmental Protection Agency (EPA) and the Occupational Safety and Health Administration (OSHA) provide regulation and guidelines as to how hazardous materials are handled.

Hazardous materials in the medical environment can include biological, chemical, radiological, and physical hazards. Biological hazardous materials are commonly referred to as **biohazards**. These are materials that present a threat to the health of living things, primarily humans. Biohazards are typically introduced into the medical environment in the form of patient body fluids and excreta. Examples of biohazardous materials are blood, body fluids, viruses, and bacteria. Items in the medical environment that have been exposed to biohazardous materials are considered to be biohazardous, as well, until the decontamination process is completed. For example, used surgical instruments are considered biohazardous until they have been cleaned of bioburden and sterilized.

Chemical hazardous materials in the medical environment include solid, liquid, or gas materials that pose a threat to health. Primarily, solid and liquid chemical hazards include materials used to clean, disinfect, and sanitize the medical environment. They may also include cytotoxic and chemotherapy medications. Gas chemicals are primarily anesthetic gases. Containers for chemical hazards are labeled with symbols representing the type of potential hazard, along with instructions for steps to take in the event of exposure.

Radiological hazards found in the medical environment are seen in the forms of thermal, radioactive isotopes, and electromagnetic radiation. The most common thermal radiological hazard is in the form of laser. The use of lasers exposes the patient and the health care team to risk of eye damage, as well as increasing the risk of fire in the operating room. Laser operators must be trained on the correct usage of the laser, along with indicated safety precautions. Radioactive isotopes are used in brachytherapy. **Brachytherapy** is a form of cancer treatment where radioactive beads are inserted near or inside a cancerous tumor in order to deliver a high dose of radiation to the tumor while sparing the surrounding healthy tissue. Electromagnetic radiation is seen in the form of x-ray and ultraviolet radiation. During a procedure where electromagnetic radiation is used, the patient is protected by shields and/or drapes specifically designed to minimize exposure to the radiation. The perioperative team utilizes shields, gowns, and eyewear to minimize radiation exposure.

Physical hazards also exist in the medical area. **Autoclaves** are used to steam sterilize surgical instruments, and this steam can potentially cause burns. Removing surgical instruments straight from the autoclave can cause burns to the hands if the proper gloves are not used. Liquid on the floor can cause someone to slip or fall, causing injury. Handling carbon dioxide tanks or cryogenic material can cause severe burns to the hands if gloves are not worn.

The types of hazards should be discussed at the beginning of employment in the medical environment. This should include identifying the potential hazards and known hazards, steps to minimize exposure to them, and discussing the necessary steps to take in case of exposure. Healthcare facilities are required to provide materials safety data sheets (MSDS) and keep them in a central area. For most healthcare facilities, education on hazardous materials management is done on an annual basis.

Comfort Measures and Patient Responses

Spirituality

Spirituality may play a positive role in patients' coping response. **Spirituality** refers to a personal understanding and acceptance of one's role and meaning in the grand scheme of existence. It can be religious, faith-based, an energetic understanding, or a simple, personal reflection. This can be another dimension for healthcare providers to investigate and utilize with patients as they prepare them for a surgical procedure or help them recover. Patients who have a strong spiritual practice of any sort are associated with having more peaceful responses to their personal health, higher levels of stress control, less pain after surgical procedures, and easier recovery periods after medical procedures.

Psychological Response

Thoughts and emotions have a significant role in the concept of medical procedures. Patients may have psychologic distress such as depression and anxiety. Because some psychiatric syndromes are interpreted by self-reported pain, patients who are unable to accurately describe their pain are mistakenly assumed to have a psychiatric disorder, which in turn denies them of proper care. Pain impairs attention, memory, concentration, and content of thought.

Preparation of the Surgical Site

Anatomy and Physiology

Anatomical and physiological information that is relevant to a patient's case is essential in order for adequate and effective perioperative nursing care to take place. Before a procedure, nursing staff should understand the anatomical functioning of the operation site in order to prepare the patient for the procedure and recovery. For example, a patient who is undergoing a lung procedure will have different operative and recovery needs (based on the function of respiration) than a patient who is undergoing a foot surgery (who will have needs based on the function of walking).

Skin Prep Antisepsis

The skin is an important front-line defense of the body in protecting it against infectious pathogens. Sterilizing the skin is not possible, but steps can be taken by the perioperative nurse to decrease the chance of surgical site infection. **Skin prep antisepsis** can be broken down into three objectives: remove the soil, debris, and transient microorganisms from the skin surface; reduce the number of resident microorganisms on the skin; and inhibit rebound microorganism growth on the skin. Removing any soil and debris on the skin is the first step in skin prep antisepsis. This can be achieved by using alcohol wipes to remove skin oils, or even using soap, water, and a washcloth to wash the skin. Some transient microorganisms can be removed by this process, also. Transient microorganisms are those that the skin has been exposed to from an external source. After removing soil and debris, the skin should be allowed to dry before proceeding to the next phase of skin prep antisepsis.

The second objective of skin prep antisepsis is to reduce the number of resident microorganisms on the skin. Resident microorganisms are those that are present as part of the flora of the patient. Perspiration raises these microorganisms from the deeper skin levels to the skin surface. Removal of hair at the area of planned surgical incision is another step-in skin prep. Hair contains microorganisms that remain in place, even after the skin prep antisepsis process. Because this increases the risk of surgical site infection, best practice guidelines recommend removing hair at the surgical site. Hair should be removed using a clipper with a single-use clipper blade. Using a razor is not recommended, because a razor can break the skin and increase infection risk.

After visible soil and debris are cleansed from the skin and hair is removed from the surgical site, a skin prep solution is used to reduce the resident microbial skin count and inhibit rebound growth of microorganisms. The type of skin prep solution used depends on the type of surgical procedure, as well as the policy of the healthcare institution. The two most commonly used prep solutions are chlorhexidine gluconate and povidone iodine. Evidence-based practice guidelines suggest chlorhexidine gluconate can be more effective in reducing surgical site infection rates, and many institutions have policies that dictate using chlorhexidine gluconate, unless contraindicated. Chlorhexidine gluconate is a widely used antiseptic that decreases microbial counts of the skin, mucosa, and oral cavity. In surgical skin prep antisepsis, chlorhexidine gluconate is available in alcohol-based skin scrub prep, oral rinse, and soap.

For intraoperative skin prep antisepsis, a solution of chlorhexidine gluconate and isopropyl alcohol is routinely used. ChloraPrep is an example of this type of solution. It is widely used as the preferred skin prep antisepsis solution. Because it is an alcohol-based scrub prep, it must be allowed to completely dry prior to applying surgical drapes. Failure to allow it to dry can result in pooling of solution under the skin and on the surgical drapes. Since alcohol is an ignition source, this increases the risk of surgical fire in the presence of electrosurgical unit cautery. Chlorhexidine gluconate prep is contraindicated in patients with chlorhexidine allergy. Alcohol-based prep is contraindicated on broken skin, mucous membranes (including eyes and genitourinary areas), and pediatric patients. Povidone-iodine is a broad-spectrum antiseptic for topical use.

Povidone-iodine can be used as a scrub prep or paint prep. Since it is not alcohol-based, it is safe to use on broken skin and mucous membranes. It is contraindicated in patients with an allergy to iodine.

Regardless of the type of solution used for skin prep antisepsis, the perioperative nurse should be versed in the indications and contraindications for use, as well as the manufacturer guidelines for use.

Selection of Procedure-Specific Barrier Materials

Invasive procedures increase the risk of infection in patients. Intentional incisions created by the surgical instruments can facilitate the introduction of microorganisms into the patient's tissues. Strict infection control practices are crucial throughout the perioperative experience to prevent complications.

Barriers utilized pre and intraoperatively help decrease the risk of infection. The types of barriers used are dependent on the scheduled procedure. Preoperatively, the main barriers used to prevent infection are antimicrobial skin antiseptic solutions, specifically products containing chlorhexidine gluconate (CHG). Patients should be instructed to shower or bathe before the procedure with a CHG soap or solution. Special attention must be given to the area that will be exposed during the procedure. A three-step process of applying, lathering, and rinsing should be emphasized. Patients who are unable to bathe themselves should be assisted or given a bed bath with CHG microfiber cloths. The application of antiseptic solution leaves a film on the skin that acts as an initial barrier to microorganisms.

Surgical draping is one of the primary methods of intraoperative infection control. Surgical drapes are manufactured in various sizes and shapes to cover equipment, furniture, and the patient. A drape provides a physical barrier between the patient and microbes in the environment, thus decreasing the risk of infection. Drapes may be disposable, in the form of paper, or reusable cloths with appropriate sanitizing protocols.

The type of drape used is dependent on the anatomical location for the procedure. For example, a fenestrated drape is used when surgeries are to be performed on the abdomen, flank, or thoracic cavity. The fenestration (or window) allows for isolated exposure to the site. Other drapes allow enough room for the procedure to be performed while still providing a barrier to the rest of the body, such as abdominal or orthopedic drapes. Clear drapes are placed on surgical instruments and equipment, such as the da Vinci robot for laparotomies or a camera for endoscopic procedures. The clear drapes provide a barrier between the surgical instrument and the patient's body cavity.

Personal protective equipment such as gloves, gowns, masks, face shields, goggles, and shoe and hair covers are standard in the operating room. These barriers provide protection from microbes to the operating room staff as well as the patient. Additional equipment may be required for specific patients. For example, a procedure performed on a patient with tuberculosis requires specific airborne ventilation to prevent environmental contamination. These rooms require negative airflow to contain air particles within the operating room.

Barriers applied postoperatively help protect the patient from infection and injury. The type of protective barrier is dependent on the type of procedure performed. For example, a patient who had surgery to the eye will require a protective eye shield to prevent accidental injury. Patients treated surgically for burns may have antimicrobial ointments applied as a barrier to infection in the postoperative period.

Patient Responses to Pharmacological Agents

Most of the nurse's day-to-day work will involve the administration of pharmacological and parenteral therapies as part of the pain management side of the patient's treatment plan. In general,

pharmacological therapy has to do with the branch of science in which drugs are created for the use of combatting disease processes. Each of these drugs is administered into the body via pill, patch, or otherwise and has a measurable, desired effect on the body. Parenteral therapies are a specific mode of medication delivery via some other route than the alimentary canal, usually by a needle. This can be intravenous (IV), intrathecal, intraosseous, and subcutaneous, among other routes.

With all medication administration, the nurse must be mindful of the drug's potential adverse effects. As far as pharmacology has come in the past century, no drug has been perfected to the point of not having any potential adverse effect. An **adverse effect** is defined as a negative response to a medication that is not part of the desired effect. The chemical structure of the drug is what usually triggers these adverse effects. Adverse effects are greatly minimized by appropriate dosing for the individual patient.

Some drug side effects are quite obvious. Take, for example, warfarin. Warfarin, or Coumadin, is used to thin out the blood in patients at risk for forming deadly blood clots, such as those with atrial fibrillation. However, if inappropriately dosed and under-monitored, warfarin can cause serious hemorrhaging because of its effect on the body's clotting mechanisms and ability to achieve hemostasis. Patients taking warfarin should be carefully monitored for overdosage and signs of bleeding.

At times, a drug may cause an adverse effect when it is co-administered with some other substance that affects its chemical structure or its ability to be absorbed by the body. Narcotics, for example, should not be taken while drinking alcohol. Alcohol, a depressant, exacerbates the effect of the narcotic, also a depressant, to the point that the patient's drive to breathe and their consciousness may be completely knocked out, causing death.

Another type of adverse effect is an allergic reaction. Depending on the patient's unique immune system's makeup, some drugs may cause the immune system to kick into overdrive, decreasing the desired effect and adding a lot of unwanted effects. Common signs of an allergic reaction include mild reactions such as itching and rash, escalating all the way to a severe reaction such as anaphylactic shock. **Anaphylaxis** involves an inflammation and narrowing of the patient's airway. This makes breathing difficult and presents a life-threatening situation.

The nurse should be aware of common contraindications for a certain drug's use. A **contraindication** is a situation in which it is inappropriate to administer a drug. For example, if a patient is taking a potassium-sparing ACE inhibitor for the management of heart failure, supplementation of potassium should be avoided or only carefully done under the management of the attending physician or nephrologist. This is because the ACE inhibitor causes the body to excrete *less* potassium than it normally does, meaning supplementing potassium puts the patient at risk for hyperkalemia, a life-threatening condition that can cause heart rhythm abnormalities and dysfunction. Another common contraindication to be mindful of is the administration of Coumadin, or warfarin, with another blood thinner such as aspirin. The concurrent usage of these two medications aimed at decreasing the body's own hemostatic response can result in a life-threatening hemorrhage in the patient and should be avoided.

If the nurse ever suspects that the administration of a drug is contraindicated by the usage of another, they should always raise their concern with the ordering physician, the pharmacist on staff, and/or nursing management to confirm. It is a patient safety issue that is worth the extra time to investigate to prevent patient harm.

Adverse effects and contraindications are some of the rarer occurrences in day-to-day pharmacological therapies that the nurse will encounter. More commonly, the nurse will encounter milder, unwanted effects of drug administration called **side effects**. Most drugs have side effects or undesirable effects of administration. For example, a patient put on antibiotics for a respiratory infection may experience gastrointestinal (GI) upset such as stomachache, excessive flatulence, and diarrhea. Antibiotics destroy the native GI tract bacteria as part of their mechanism of action, which is what causes these side effects. Side effects are usually mild enough that the patient can either bear with them until they are finished taking the medication for the original cause, or the doctor may prescribe a counter drug to lessen the side effects of the original drug. As each additional drug carries with it the potential for more side effects, use of more medications should be weighed carefully as to their potential for helping the patient. The clinical judgment of the doctor and nurse and the patient's preference are all considered in these decisions.

Drug interactions are an aspect of pharmacology that the nurse must keep in mind when performing medication administration. A **drug interaction** may occur between many different drugs and substances. These interactions may fall into one of three categories: synergistic, antagonistic, or an interaction in which a whole new action is produced that neither substance could produce on their own.

A **synergistic interaction** is one in which the two concurrently administered substances *enhance* each other's action. Sometimes the prescriber uses the synergistic action of drugs to their advantage when the synergy would be helpful to the patient's condition. In some instances, however, synergy of two drugs is detrimental to the patient. An example of synergistic medications working in the patient's best interest would be the use of multiple antibiotics to treat an infection. Many patients with respiratory infections, such as pneumonia, will be prescribed a combination of different antibiotic therapies for two reasons. One is that the prescriber does not always know the exact causative organism of the infection and wants to wipe it out completely, and two, these combinations of antibiotics have been shown to be more effective than just using one specific antibiotic.

An example of synergistic drugs having an unwanted effect is the combination of multiple blood thinners, such as Coumadin and aspirin, that was mentioned above. In some patients' cases, the combination of the two drugs may be warranted and helpful, while in others it could have a devastating effect on the patient, resulting in a massive bleed.

Antagonistic drug interactions are ones in which the two co-administered substances cancel each other out or greatly decrease each other's potential action. Patients who are taking cholesterol-lowering drugs such as statins, for example, are discouraged from drinking grapefruit juice, as it has an antagonistic action on the statin. The grapefruit essentially absorbs all the statins before the body can, thus canceling out any positive effects they might have had for the patient, rendering them useless.

A nurse who is well versed in pharmacological knowledge, including drug side effects, adverse effects, contraindications, and interactions, will be able to better serve and protect their patients from harm.

Anesthesia Management

Perioperative anesthesia may be administered by an anesthesiologist or a **certified registered nurse anesthetist (CRNA)**. Depending on the practice setting, the perioperative nurse may administer certain intravenous moderate sedation medications and provide moderate sedation monitoring. The type of anesthesia is selected after patient assessment, history and physical, and diagnostic tests. Other factors that determine the type of anesthesia used are patient preference, age, length of surgery, surgeon preference, and the **American Society of Anesthesiologists (ASA)** classification.

ASA classification is a method of assessing patient health status prior to surgery. The patient is given an ASA value of I through VI:

- ASA I indicates a healthy patient. The ASA I patient is at low risk for complications based on health status.
- ASA II is given to a patient with mild systemic disease. Pregnancy, obesity, controlled diabetes, and controlled hypertension put the patient into ASA II status.
- The patient with severe systemic disease that is not incapacitating is an ASA III. Patients with uncontrolled diabetes, poorly managed hypertension, chronic obstructive pulmonary disease (COPD), end stage renal disease (ESRD), remote history of cerebrovascular accident (CVA), or remote history of myocardial infarction (MI) can be classified as ASA III.
- ASA IV indicates the patient has severe systemic disease that is a constant threat to life. Examples of this are recent history of MI or CVA, cardiac ischemia, significant heart valve dysfunction, and ejection fraction below twenty percent.
- ASA V describes the patient who is near death and is not expected to survive without the operation. The patient with a ruptured abdominal aortic aneurysm (AAA), acute cardiac tamponade, or intracranial bleed can be categorized as ASA V.
- The patient who has been declared brain dead and is being kept alive for the purpose of organ recovery is classified as ASA VI. In addition to ASA classes I through VI, the procedure is given an "E" after the class designation if it is an emergency procedure. The patient with a ruptured abdominal aortic aneurysm can be designated an ASA "VE."

There are three types of anesthesia: general, regional, and local. General anesthesia consists of amnesia, analgesia, and muscle relaxation. With general anesthesia, the patient is unconscious and needs cardiopulmonary support. This support usually includes the placement of an endotracheal tube (ETT) or laryngeal mask airway (LMA) for airway management. General anesthesia is broken down into three phases: induction, maintenance, and emergence. The induction phase is from administration of anesthetic agent until surgical incision. The maintenance phase is from surgical incision until the end of the surgical procedure, or until the near end of the procedure. Emergence begins when the patient begins to awaken and ends when the patient leaves the operating room. If an ETT or LMA is present, it can be removed during emergence if the patient is supporting their own airway and is breathing adequately.

Medications used in general anesthesia may include intravenous agents, inhalation gases, and muscle relaxants. Intravenous agents used for induction include thiopental, propofol, ketamine, and etomidate. Benzodiazepines, including midazolam and valium, may be administered in conjunction with induction agents to achieve amnesia. Inhalation gases are often used in pediatric patient to induce anesthesia prior to placement of intravenous catheter. Inhalation gases used in induction are nitrous oxide and sevoflurane. Isoflurane and desflurane are anesthetic gases used primarily for maintenance of anesthesia. Muscle relaxants are indicated in certain surgical procedures. Ventilator support must be provided if muscle relaxants are used, since these medications act as paralytics. Succinylcholine and rocuronium are commonly used muscle relaxants.

Regional anesthesia is achieved when local anesthetic is injected along a nerve pathway. Regional anesthesia may be used alone or in combination with moderate sedation. Regional anesthesia is a good option for patients who are deemed too high risk for undergoing general anesthesia. Types of regional anesthesia are spinal, epidural, and Bier block.

Spinal anesthesia is achieved when anesthetic is injected directly into the spinal canal. The effects of spinal anesthesia depend on where in the spinal column the medication is injected. Spinal anesthesia may be used in caesarean sections or in lower extremity revascularizations. Complications of spinal anesthesia include severe hypotension, respiratory compromise, and headache.

Epidural anesthesia is achieved by injecting anesthetic into the epidural space. Epidural anesthesia may be administered as a single dose or as an infusion via catheter placement into the epidural space. Epidural anesthesia may be used in caesarean sections, as well as for postoperative pain management for thoracotomies. Complications of epidural anesthesia include dural puncture and intravascular injection.

A Bier block is often used for upper extremity nerve blockade. It is achieved by applying a tourniquet to the upper extremity, raising the arm to promote drainage of blood away from the arm, inflating the tourniquet, and then applying local anesthetic to the area distal to the tourniquet. The local anesthetic remains in the surgical area until the tourniquet is slowly deflated, in order to not release a bolus of local anesthetic into circulation.

Local anesthesia may be used in healthy patients or in those unable to tolerate general anesthesia. Local anesthetic agents such as lidocaine and bupivacaine act at the injection site and do not alter the patient's mental status. Local anesthetics may be used alone or in combination with intravenous analgesics, such as fentanyl. Midazolam may also be used to achieve amnesic effect. In monitored anesthesia care (MAC), the patient receives local anesthetic along with sedation and analgesia. The goals of MAC are safe patient sedation, pain control, and anxiety control. The patient undergoing conscious sedation with MAC is able to answer questions, support their own airway, and follow commands.

Cricoid Pressure

Cricoid pressure is a safe practice utilized in intraoperative care when rapid sequence intubation is required. The technique is most commonly practiced in emergency surgeries. In these cases, patients are not scheduled for the surgery and therefore have not taken the necessary preoperative precautions, such as fasting. Any gastrointestinal contents present the risk of regurgitation into the lungs and consequent asphyxiation when the patient is anesthetized. The application of pressure at the location of cricoid tissue creates an internal esophageal seal, blocking the pathway to the lungs and mitigating asphyxiation risk. Intubation occurs after this takes place.

Seven Rights

The "seven rights" refer to a set of seven guidelines for healthcare providers to follow when administering medication to patients. These standardize the medication administration process and promote a context of high quality care. The seven rights are:

- Right medication: Providers check that the medication they are about to administer is the one that was prescribed.
- Right client: Providers check that the patient who is about to receive medication is the correct patient.
- Right dose: Providers check that the dose they are about to administer matches the prescribed dose.
- Right time: Providers check that the medication is given at the pre-determined interval.
- Right route: Providers ensure that medication is delivered in the intended method (e.g., orally).
- Right reason: Providers note that the medication is administered for a specific cause.
- Right documentation: Providers follow institutional protocol to maintain thorough recordkeeping of administered medications.

Medication Management

Intraoperative medications are managed by the anesthesiologist, circulating nurse, and the surgical field. The anesthesiologist manages and administers intravenous anesthetics and anesthetic gases, medications for hemodynamic management, and antibiotics during the intraoperative period. The anesthesiologist assesses the patient's response to the medications by monitoring electrocardiogram (ECG), **blood pressure**, and **end tidal carbon dioxide (ETCO2)**. The anesthesiologist documents the name, dosage, route, and time of medication in the medical record.

The circulating nurse documents all medications administered to the patient from the surgical field. These medications include antibiotic irrigation, hemostasis agents, vasodilators, local anesthetics, and thrombolytic agents. The circulating nurse documents the name, dose, route, and time of medication administration in the medical record. If the patient is receiving procedural sedation by a perioperative nurse, the sedation nurse manages, administers, and documents all medications administered to the patient, excluding those administered from the surgical field.

In addition to documentation of all medications administered intraoperatively, medication management includes labeling and storing medication according to guidelines set by regulating bodies and institutional policies. All medications on the surgical field must be labeled with the name and strength of the medication clearly visible. This includes any fluids on the surgical field. In labeling medications, approved abbreviations must be used. For instance, a basin containing normal saline is labeled with a sticker on the basin that reads *0.9% NaCl* or *Normal Saline*. Since *NS* is not an approved abbreviation for normal saline, the medication label should not read *NS*. Syringes on the surgical field must also be clearly labeled, identifying the medication name and strength.

Medications off the surgical field are also labeled. This includes IV tubing and infusion bags, multi-dose medication vials, and medication syringes with medication not immediately used. For example, if the anesthesiologist draws up medication from a single-use medication vial and performs another task prior to administering the medication, the medication in the syringe must be labeled with medication name and strength. This is a patient safety issue.

Narcotic medication management has its own set of guidelines, including distribution and documentation of narcotic usage. The potential for narcotic abuse guides strict documentation of narcotic chain of custody. Most institutions use a central form of medication dispensing, such as a Pyxis system. Pyxis is managed by the institutional pharmacy and is stocked by pharmacists and pharmacy technicians. Access to Pyxis is granted to those approved to remove and use the medications; generally, nurses and anesthesiologists.

When a narcotic is removed from this system, the narcotic count is verified by the person removing the narcotic, and the narcotic is then removed and administered to the patient. If the person initiating narcotic removal discovers an incorrect narcotic count, the Pyxis system shows the last transaction involving the medication, including the name of the person who removed it and the prior narcotic count. The discrepancy must be resolved at that point, or the issue is turned over to pharmacy and/or hospital security. If a narcotic is removed from the system and the full dose is not administered to the patient, the narcotic must be wasted with another licensed person (such as nurse or anesthesiologist) witnessing the waste. This is documented either on paper or in the Pyxis system.

Environmental Factors

Components of the perioperative environment are regulated according to evidence-based guidelines supporting infection control and patient safety. Examples of perioperative **environmental factors** are room temperature, humidity, air exchange patterns, noise, and room traffic. Healthcare institutions create policies around each of these to guide optimal perioperative patient care practices. These policies are typically guided from AORN standards.

The recommended room temperature (according to AORN) is between sixty-eight and seventy-five degrees Fahrenheit. Temperatures below sixty-eight degrees can lead to patient hypothermia, which increases risk of surgical site infection (SSI). Conversely, temperatures above seventy-five degrees compromise the comfort level of perioperative team members, particularly those scrubbed in at the surgical field. Perioperative room temperatures are recorded daily. If the room temperature is adjusted out of the acceptable range outlined in the healthcare facility policy, the surgeon documents this into the patient medical record, along with the indication for temperature adjustment. For instance, if the patient undergoes cardiopulmonary circulatory arrest, the patient condition warrants the room temperature to be colder, in addition to other patient cooling measures. For the patient in sickle-cell crisis, the patient condition calls for a warmer room and additional patient warming measures.

The humidity level of the perioperative environment is controlled to decrease risk of SSI and to promote comfort of the perioperative team. Humidity levels in the operating room are generally between twenty and sixty percent. Keeping the humidity level below sixty percent inhibits bacterial growth within the patient and on inanimate objects within the environment, such as surgical instruments. Comfort of the perioperative team is also an important consideration. If the surgeon is uncomfortable, keeping focused can be more difficult. This increases the risk of surgeon error and compromises patient safety.

Proper air flow in the perioperative environment is essential for infection control. The recommendation for air in and out of the operating room is twenty-five air volume exchanges per hour. Air volume exchanges help to rid the air of any airborne particles. Any area that supports a sterile environment (operating room, sterile hallway, or sterile core) is maintained with a positive air pressure to facilitate the movement of particles out of the sterile area.

Noise in the perioperative environment should be kept to a minimum. This decreases the chance for distraction of the perioperative team and promotes patient safety. One way to control noise levels is to avoid unnecessary conversations and keep voices low. Having only the necessary team members in the operating room helps in controlling noise levels. If two or three side conversations are happening, the surgeon can potentially become distracted and frustrated, compromising patient safety.

Traffic in and out of the operating room should be kept to necessary traffic only. When traffic in and out of the room is necessary, the door leading into the sterile hallway should be used. The door leading into the nonsterile hallway should be avoided in order to preserve the sterile atmosphere in the operating room.

Infectious Waste

Infectious waste refers to waste that occurs during medical examination, treatment, autopsy, or some other procedure relating to human or animal tissues, bodily fluids, or bone. Infectious waste includes items such as blood, plasma, fecal or urine matter, bacterial or viral cultures, materials used in surgery or recovery, pharmaceuticals, syringes, and so on. This type of waste must be handled differently from traditional waste due to its infectious and pathogenic nature. In the medical setting, it must be collected separately from other types of waste and marked as such. Infectious waste is then removed from the building and sterilized at an external facility before it is landfilled or recycled.

Maintaining a Sterile Field

Aseptic and Sterile Technique

In discussing **aseptic technique**, it is important to know the difference between the terms "aseptic" and "sterile." The term aseptic refers to the absence of pathogenic microorganisms, and sterile means the absence of all microorganisms. Aseptic technique is essential in maintaining sterility of the operating room environment. When discussing **sterile technique**, it is important to note the principles of sterile technique.

The **Association of perioperative Registered Nurses (AORN)** has published eight recommendations for sterile technique practices:

- Recommendation I addresses the need for perioperative personnel to implement practices designed to reduce transmission of infectious organisms when working in an operative or invasive procedure environment. Best practice guidelines for surgical attire and hand hygiene fall under this recommendation. Aseptic principles are applied in conjunction with sterile technique to reduce the risk of contamination of the sterile field, and ultimately, reduce the risk of adverse events related to the introduction of pathogens into the sterile field. Aseptic and sterile technique practices are designed to optimize wound healing and prevent surgical site infection.

- Recommendation II speaks to the selection of surgical gowns, gloves, and drapes using evidence-based guidelines. These products should be selected for safety and efficacy prior to use. Many organizations have product-selection committees that focus on choosing safe, cost-effective supplies.

- Recommendation III refers to the use of sterile technique in donning a sterile gown and gloves. The members of the surgical team who perform in a scrubbed role perform surgical skin antisepsis prior to donning sterile gloves and gowns. Sterile gowns and gloves are worn by all scrubbed-in team members. The sterile zones of the surgical gown are the front (from the chest to the level of the sterile field) and at the sleeves from two inches above the elbow to the sleeve cuff.

- Recommendation IV focuses on the use of sterile drapes and the proper placement of them. Choosing the proper type of drape for the type of surgery being performed is also highlighted. A drape with a small surgical field opening, such as a thyroid drape, is ideal for a procedure where the incision area is small. Cesarean section drapes have clear plastic pockets on the sides that are designed to contain amniotic fluid after the incision into the uterus.

- In Recommendation V, the use of a sterile field in surgical and invasive procedures is laid out. Sterile items should only be used within a sterile field. After sterile items are introduced to a nonsterile environment, they are no longer considered sterile. When the sterility of an item is questionable, consider the item to be contaminated. When in doubt, throw it out. Sterile team members must only touch sterile surfaces, and nonsterile members only touch nonsterile surfaces. Tables within the sterile field are considered sterile at tabletop level, but not below it. The edges of sterile tables and trays are considered unsterile.

- Recommendation VI addresses opening sterile supplies onto the sterile field, as well as how to assess the integrity of the sterile field. A sterile item is contained within a sterile barrier. If this barrier is compromised in any way, the item is no longer sterile. For example, if a sterile instrument's impervious surgical wrap has a tear in it, the instrument is considered contaminated.

- Recommendation VII addresses best practice for monitoring of the sterile field and how to address a breach of sterile technique. The sterile field must be constantly monitored. As long as the sterile field is monitored, it will last the duration of the surgical procedure. This is true even if the procedure lasts several hours. An unmonitored sterile field, however, is no longer a sterile field.

- Recommendation VIII addresses how to monitor movement within and around the sterile field. Movement around the sterile field must not be done in a manner that contaminates the field. Nonsterile team members should remain at least twelve inches away from the sterile field. Nonsterile objects should not reach over the sterile field. This includes the arm of the nonsterile circulating nurse opening sterile objects onto the sterile field. Nonsterile persons should not walk in between two sterile fields.

Infection Prevention and Control

Surgical Site Infections Risk Factors

Patient Factors

- Age
- Diabetes
- Nicotine or Steroid Use
- Altered Immune Response
- Malnutrition or Obesity
- Preoperative colonization with Staph. aureus
- Prolonged Preoperative Stay

Infection prevention and control are paramount objectives in providing safe healthcare. Patients in the perioperative environment are at increased risk of hospital-acquired infection (HAI) as compared to those not undergoing surgery. The surgical incision creates a way for pathogens to be introduced into the body. Evidence-based guidelines for prevention of surgical site infection (SSI) are adopted by all accredited healthcare institutions.

Measures in prevention of SSI are laid out by organizations such as the **Centers for Disease Control and Prevention (CDC)**, the Institute for Healthcare Improvement (IHI), and The Joint Commission (TJC). Infection prevention and control must be viewed from a multifactorial viewpoint in perioperative nursing. Standard precautions are used in the perioperative setting as a method to reduce infection rates. Standard precautions include hand hygiene, the use of **personal protective equipment (PPE)**, and environmental control.

In all healthcare settings, the gold standard in infection prevention is hand hygiene. Hand hygiene includes consistency in hand washing and antisepsis at the correct times and with the proper technique. Although hand hygiene is known to be a simple, effective way to prevent the spread of infectious pathogens (including **multi-drug resistant organisms [MDROs]**), the CDC reports healthcare providers clean their hands less than one half of the times they should.

Healthcare providers use PPE as a way to protect themselves from being exposed to infectious material from the patient and healthcare environment. PPE used in the perioperative setting includes surgical masks, gloves, eye shields, impervious gowns, and shoe covers. PPE is also utilized in patient resuscitation with the use of a bag-valve mask or ambu bag rather than mouth-to-mouth resuscitation. Environmental control is an important aspect of infection prevention, because it decreases transmission of pathogens from environmental surfaces to patients and/or healthcare workers. Using approved disinfectants according to manufacturer instructions is an effective environmental control measure in infection control and prevention.

When a patient is colonized or infected with a known MDRO, transmission-based precautions are taken. Transmission-based precautions are used along with standard precautions. The three categories of transmission-based precautions are contact, droplet, and airborne. The indication depends on the MDRO.

Contact precautions are used with patients infected or colonized with microorganisms transmitted by direct or indirect contact. These include *Clostridium difficile* (*C. diff*), methicillin resistant *Staphylococcus aureus* (MRSA), and vancomycin resistant *Enterococcus* (VRE).

Droplet precautions are used if a patient has a confirmed or suspected infection transmissible through respiratory droplets. PPE associated with droplet precautions are gloves, gown, and mask. The patient is also placed in a single-patient room. Influenza and respiratory syncytial virus (RSV) are indications for droplet precautions.

Airborne precautions are taken when providing care to a patient with known or suspected infection transmissible via airborne route. The patient's respiratory particles are airborne for prolonged time periods and are carried by normal air currents. The most common airborne-transmissible infections are tuberculosis, measles, and varicella.

Central line associated bloodstream infection (CLABSI) prevention begins at the time of central line insertion. Often, central lines are inserted in the operating room. CLABSI bundles are used in an effort to reduce CLABSI. These bundles vary, but generally include steps to ensure proper skin prep, sterile technique, initial central line dressing, guidelines for subsequent dressing changes, and recommendations for removing central line as soon as possible. Catheter-associated urinary tract infection (CAUTI) is another consideration for infection risk in the perioperative patient population. One initiative in preventing CAUTI is inserting urinary catheters only in patients who meet certain criteria. Commonly, these criteria are surgery of the genitourinary tract, anticipated long operative time (greater than a couple of hours), risk of urine entering the sterile field, need for intraoperative urinary output monitoring, and need for core temperature monitoring. Extended presence of a urinary catheter is also associated with CAUTI, so discontinuing the urinary catheter as soon as possible decreases the risk of CAUTI.

Protecting Patients' Dignity, Privacy, and Rights

Patient Rights and Responsibilities

Patients have rights and responsibilities when it comes to their health care. Generally, these are communicated to the patient in a Patient's Bill of Rights document at the entry point of care. Safety is an inherent patient right and expectation. Patients have the right to be informed on their disease process, treatment plan, and alternatives to treatment. Patient and family education should be included during the nursing process. In addition, the patient has the right to be involved in decisions involving their care. A patient may access their medical record upon request by following the process set by the health care facility. HIPAA protects patient rights around confidentiality, release of medical information, and privacy.

All patients have the right to affordable, quality care based upon best practices, regardless of ability to pay. Patients should be cared for in a respectful, nondiscriminatory fashion. Patients have the right to comfort measures, as well as pharmacological pain management (if ordered by a physician) provided in a manner that is safe. Patients who are hospitalized have the right to visitors during times allowed by the facility. Evidence-based practice supports open family visitation hours, even in critical care units. Several facilities have adopted policies supporting this practice. As previously stated, the patient has the right to respectful treatment; however, the patient is responsible for being respectful to caregivers. The patient should have a clear understanding of their rights, and health care providers are bound to do everything possible to uphold these. With that being said, the patient should be clearly informed of their responsibilities and be compliant with them.

It is important for the patient to keep scheduled appointments and arrive in a timely manner. If the patient's demographic information changes, the health provider's office should be updated in order to keep the lines of communication open. The patient is responsible for copays, deductibles, and any other fees that align with the health insurance or benefit plan. If the patient is unable to pay, they are responsible for negotiating a payment plan or deferral. If an advance directive exists, the patient must communicate this and provide a copy for health providers. The patient should actively participate in care, asking questions when necessary. To ensure appropriate care is provided, the patient must provide accurate and complete health information to providers; this includes disclosing all medications that are currently being taken. If the patient is prescribed medications, the patient is responsible for keeping medications to self only, not allowing others access to them. When the patient and health provider(s) create a plan of care, the patient should verbalize understanding of it and accept any consequences of decisions made. The patient must also be responsible for following up on instructions as directed.

Patient Advocacy

Advocacy is a key component of nursing practice. An **advocate** is one who pleads the cause of another; and the nurse is an advocate for patient rights. Preserving human dignity, patient equality, and freedom from suffering are the basis of nursing advocacy. Nurses hold a significant role that gives them the opportunity to care for patients in every way: caring for their needs, addressing any and all concerns, and ensuring that all outcomes are positive. More experienced nurses can aid in communicating with doctors and physicians while also serving as a guide through the complexities of the medical system. Nurses educate the patient about tests and procedures and are aware of how culture and ethnicity affect the patient's experience. Nurses strictly adhere to all privacy laws.

Of utmost importance in the perioperative setting is the nurse's responsibility for advocating for the patient and protecting their rights. In the OR, the patient may be under anesthesia and unable to speak for themselves, so inherently, the nurse is responsible for speaking on their behalf. Further, the patient has a right to privacy that sometimes seems a lesser priority once the patient is asleep, positioned, prepped, and draped. At all times, the perioperative nurse must ensure that they are serving as the best advocate for the patient.

Advocating for the patient may include activities like calling attention to potential or actual breaks in sterility, requesting that nonessential conversation take place after the procedure as opposed to during the procedure, or restricting the number of unnecessary visitors in the OR. When the patient is under the drapes, it can be easy to forget that on the table is a person with rights to the best available care and privacy.

Another practice that has become widely adopted is covering of windows for procedures, such as gynecological or urological procedures, where the patient may be very exposed. This provides additional privacy to the patient because personnel walking down the hallway will be prevented from observing the patient in a compromising position from outside the room. In these procedures, there is an inherent vulnerability due to the area of the body being operated on or the position the patient must be in for the procedure. Covering the window is a simple way to treat the patient with dignity and respect.

Protect Patient Confidentiality

Patient privacy and confidentiality is a constant for all health care providers. Given the sensitivity of surgical procedures, the perioperative team must maintain strict **patient confidentiality**. Under the Health Insurance Portability and Accountability Act (HIPAA), a patient's information is required to be protected and kept confidential regardless of the form, including electronic, written, and spoken communication. Protected health information (PHI) should be shared only on an as needed and minimum necessary basis. When discussing patients or cases in settings where other personnel may overhear the conversation, the perioperative team should be careful not to include any PHI that may violate the patient's confidentiality. Additionally, when information is displayed electronically to families and visitors in waiting rooms, patient names should be avoided. HIPAA violations can have negative consequences for the providers and/or the facility.

Specimen Management

A surgical specimen is body fluid or body tissue removed from the body during the surgical procedure. The type of surgical specimen obtained depends on what lab value or tissue diagnosis is required to proceed in planning the course of patient care. Regardless of the type of specimen, standard precautions are used in handling the specimen to protect the care provider from exposure to potential hazards.

Surgical specimens include blood, urine, sputum, stool, body tissue, limbs, lymph nodes, organs, and foreign bodies. Depending on the nature of indicated testing, the surgical specimen is sent to the laboratory or pathology department for analysis. Blood, urine, sputum, and stool specimens are collected in a tube or sterile container and sent to the laboratory for testing. These tests may be ordered as stat or routine, based on the time frame for needing the results. Generally, blood tests on perioperative patients are ordered as "stat." The results are needed quickly to care for the patient effectively. Labs for routine preoperative testing, such as a urinalysis or baseline hemoglobin, are usually ordered "routine," as the results are not needed for a couple of days.

Body tissue (including organ tissue and lymph nodes) removed during surgery is considered a surgical specimen. Body tissue is often removed for diagnostic testing. In this case, the tissue is sent to the pathology department for review by the pathologist. The pathologist analyzes the tissue and makes a tissue diagnosis. The patient's course of treatment is dependent upon the tissue diagnosis. For instance, if the patient has a lung nodule suspicious of malignancy, the surgeon removes a section of lung tissue containing the nodule. This tissue is sent to the pathologist for review. The nodule is identified as having characteristics of adenocarcinoma, a type of cancer. The surgeon, using this information, consults with the patient and oncologist and develops a treatment plan.

Body parts that are surgically removed due to disease process are sent to the pathologist for analysis. This includes organ removal and limb removal. One example of necessary surgical removal of a limb is the patient with gangrene requiring an amputation to prevent systemic blood infection, or sepsis. In the case of amputation, the amputated body part is sent to pathology for analysis. The analysis report is sent to the surgeon and other physicians involved in the care of the patient. The findings generally confirm the original diagnosis and may even contain additional diagnostic information that is useful in planning the course of treatment. The pathology report is part of the patient's medical record.

If the patient presents to the operating room for removal of a foreign body, or if a foreign body is discovered during an unrelated surgery, the foreign body is sent to pathology for identification. The specimen is labeled as "foreign body" or "retained surgical item," even if the identity of the said item seems obvious. For instance, the patient with an esophageal perforation (esophageal tear or hole) may undergo surgery for placement of an esophageal stent to seal the perforation. If the surgeon discovers a thumb tack in the esophagus, the item is removed and sent to pathology labeled as "foreign body."

The post-procedure time out or post-procedure huddle should include verification of all surgical specimens with the surgeon, circulating nurse, and scrub person. This is an important step in preventing an item intended to be a surgical specimen from being discarded as waste. Care must also be taken in labeling the surgical specimen properly. Specifically, the specimen is labeled with patient name, medical record number, date and time of specimen removal, name of test(s) to be performed, and initials of the person labeling the specimen. Incorrect specimen labeling can lead to delay in patient care or entry of information into the incorrect patient record, if the name is incorrectly labeled.

Implants and Explants

The term "surgical implant" refers to an item intentionally placed inside the body during surgery that will remain in place permanently or for a specified time frame, generally longer than twenty-one days or thirty days. This time frame is defined in the healthcare institution's policies and procedures. Documentation of the surgical implant includes the implant type, manufacturer brand and lot number, serial number, location of the implant, and expiration date. This implant information is documented in the patient's medical record. The surgical department also keeps record of all implants, along with the information that is documented in the medical record. This implant log can be referenced for tracking purposes in the event of a product recall. Surgical **explants** are documented in the same fashion as implants. The type of device that is explanted, along with as much other supporting information about the explant, is recorded in the medical record and on an explant log. The explant log is kept in the same area of the surgical department as the implant log for tracking purposes.

Types of surgical implants include prosthetic heart valves, synthetic grafts, medication ports, cardiac electrical devices, joint replacements, and spinal or orthopedic plates and screws. Prosthetic heart valves may be metal or biological. Biological sources come from pig, cow, or human donors. Synthetic grafts can be made from polyester or polytetrafluoroethylene (PTFE) and may even be impregnated with a blood thinner medication called Heparin. Medication ports are implanted in patients who require long-term intravenous access for blood draws, chemotherapy, or antibiotic therapy. The port accesses the subclavian or internal jugular vein and is implanted under the skin at the subclavian area. Cardiac electrical devices include permanent pacemakers and automatic implantable cardioverter-defibrillator. These both include a generator with leads attached to the heart. Joint replacement implants are used for knee and hip replacements. These may be made of stainless steel, titanium, or polyethylene. Metal plates and screws may be used in spinal and orthopedics surgeries, such as fusions and fractures.

A surgical implant is seen as foreign matter to the body and puts the patient at risk for infection at the implant site. Strict aseptic technique should be adhered to in surgical cases involving an implant. If infection does develop, the implant is surgically removed, unless it is deemed unsafe by the surgeon to do so. Antibiotic prophylaxis is administered to patients with surgical implants to decrease the infection risk.

Verify That the Correct Implants Are Available

It is important to perform an additional preoperative verification process for patients who will require surgical implants. The nurse must be involved in the request for the implant. Based on facility protocols, the surgeon will submit a request of the specific implant for the procedure. The request must include the date of the surgery, the patient's name, the specific model to be used, and the anatomical location where the implant will be inserted. As part of the time-out protocol, it is the nurse's duty to ensure that the requested implant is available before the procedure starts. Facilities must implement a standard process for implant verification to meet regulatory requirements.

Surgical implants also contain specific tracking information, such as the manufacturer, model number, lot and serial numbers, and an expiration date if applicable. This information must be accurately documented in the patient's medical record by the circulating nurse. Because surgical implants are foreign objects that may cause complications such as allergic reactions and infections, tracking is important for product recalls and quality improvement.

Verify That the Implants Are Correctly Prepared

Before an implant can be surgically inserted into a patient, it must be prepared appropriately to decrease injury and risk of infection. The ideal implant is sterilized and individually wrapped by the manufacturer. However, not every implant will be available in this form. Healthcare facilities may need to conduct their own sterilization process before the implant can be used. Steam sterilization is the common form of disinfecting and sterilizing an implant. The implant is exposed to saturated steam under pressure. Documentation of the sterilization process is a necessary component to meet regulatory guidelines.

In the intraoperative phase, careful handling of the implant must be maintained. The circulating nurse must ensure that operating room personnel are following sterile technique when handling instruments and surgical implants. Implants must be placed on a sterile surface if patient preparation or positioning is needed before insertion. Any instrument that comes into contact with the implant must also be sterile to prevent infection. For example, a patient with a broken ankle may require hardware to stabilize the bone. The hardware must remain sterile while the skin is prepped and draped, and while the incision is made.

Prepare Explants for Final Disposition

Patients who have surgical implants may require invasive surgery to remove them, at which point it becomes an explant. Some surgical implants are permanent, while others are explanted after a certain period of time. Some surgical implants that may be removed include hip prostheses, bone stabilizing hardware, and cosmetic implants. Implants are removed when they have corrected the initial issue and are no longer warranted. The removal may also be performed due to malfunction or infection. Just as with implantation, strict documentation should accompany the procedure. Documentation should include the medical tracking information, any adverse effects that the patient experiences due to the implant, and final disposition of the surgical explant. The documentation provides pertinent information should a recall of the implant occur.

While the majority of surgical explants are returned to manufacturers or disposed of by healthcare facilities, some patients may request to obtain these postoperatively. Before an implant can be given or transported to a patient, it must be stored and handled in a manner that prevents leakage or exposure to bodily fluids. The implant is considered contaminated and must be labeled as such according to OSHA regulations. Nurses should be aware of the facility's guidelines for safe disposal of surgical explants including waste containers and possible pathology testing.

Surgical Counts

A retained surgical item is an item inadvertently left inside the patient during the surgery process. Although steps to prevent retained surgical items are included in policies and procedures of every operating facility, retentions of surgical items still occur. Because patient safety is top priority and the responsibility of the entire surgical team, it is up to every member of the surgical team to be proactive in preventing retentions of surgical items from occurring. A retained surgical item can result in the patient needing a surgical procedure to remove the item, an infection, or patient death. Aside from the patient safety implications, the financial cost of a retained surgical item is a consideration. The healthcare facility involved in a retained surgical item foots the cost of the hospitalization and surgery necessitated by the retained item. In addition, litigation resulting from the event is likely.

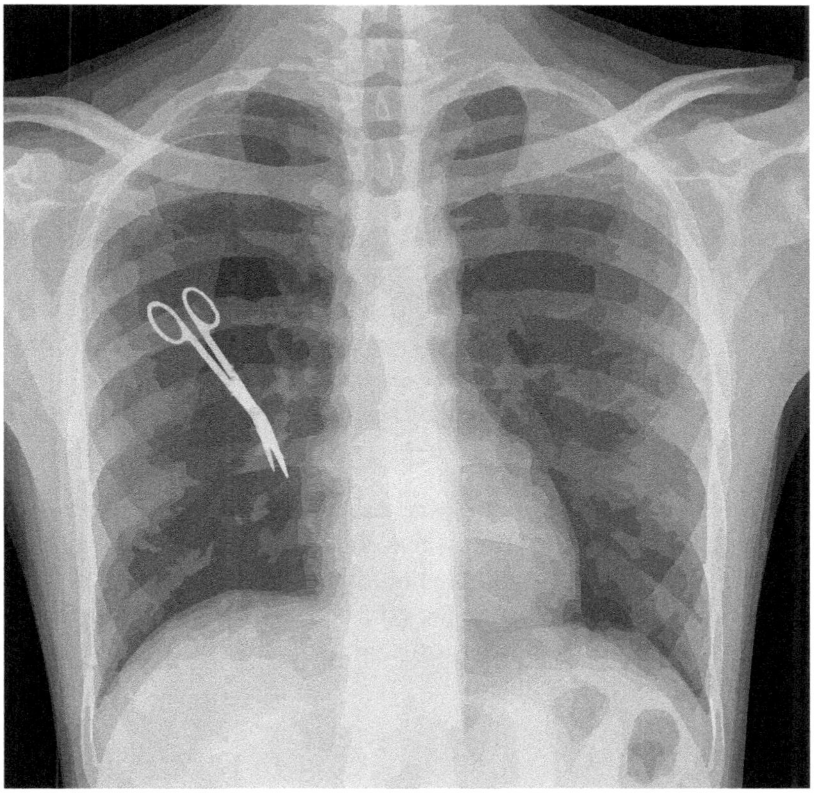

When a surgical procedure involves an incision, a surgical count must be performed to prevent items used in the procedure from being retained in the body. The surgical count involves a count of items in the surgical field prior to skin incision, a count at the beginning of closure of the body cavity or first tissue layer, and a final count during skin closure. The count of items on the surgical field must match the count inventory off the sterile field, or the count is deemed incorrect. The surgical count is performed in a two-person manner with the scrub nurse or surgical tech and the circulating nurse. Because this is a critical step in prevention of a retained surgical item, the surgical count process must not be interrupted unless absolutely necessary. For example, the circulating nurse does not stop counting to answer the telephone but stops counting to defibrillate the patient in ventricular tachycardia.

Any item that can potentially be retained in the body during surgery should be included in the surgical count. These items commonly include suture needles, hypodermic needles, surgical blades, electrosurgical cautery tips, laparotomy sponges, gauze sponges, kittners (small sponges used as blunt dissectors), tonsil sponges, and surgical towels. As a patient safety precaution, sponges and towels intended for use on the surgical field are embedded with radiography-detectable material that enables them to be seen on radiology exam (x-ray). Surgical instruments are counted in a surgical case that involves entry into a body cavity or when the potential of entry into body cavity exists, and an incision of two inches or greater is anticipated. An example of this is an open-heart procedure with a sternotomy or an abdominal procedure with entry into the peritoneal cavity. Minimally invasive cases such as a thoracoscopy or laparoscopy use incisions less than two inches for entry into a body cavity; however, the risk of converting to an "open" procedure exists. Therefore, a surgical instrument count is performed prior to skin incision.

In the event of an incorrect count, the circulating nurse informs the entire surgical team of the incorrect count and what is missing. At this point, the surgeon halts the closing process, and steps to locate the missing item are initiated. These usually involve the scrub person and circulating nurse repeating the count (to rule out a counting error), the surgeon and first assistant visually verifying the missing item is not visible at the surgical area, the anesthesiologist visually checking the area around the anesthesia machine and the surrounding floor, and the circulating nurse searching the areas off the sterile field, such as the floor or trash can. If the item is still not found, an x-ray is ordered to verify the item is not retained in the patient. The x-ray must be read and confirmed by the radiologist and communicated to the surgical team prior to the patient's leaving the operating room. If the x-ray confirms the item is not retained in the patient, the patient can continue to the next phase of care. The incorrect count and the x-ray results, along with the name of the radiologist reading the x-ray, are documented in the medical record.

The surgical count may be omitted in the event of a true emergency. If the patient presents to the emergency department with a ruptured abdominal aortic aneurysm, the surgical team must get the patient to the operating room as soon as possible in order to save the patient's life. In this case, a surgical count takes time away from life-sustaining efforts. The emergent nature of the case must be documented as the reason for omitting the surgical count, and an x-ray is performed after the procedure to verify no foreign body is retained.

Performing Universal Protocol

The Joint Commission is an agency that accredits healthcare facilities based on their regulatory compliance. The universal protocol was established by The Joint Commission to prevent an incorrect surgery or a procedure on the wrong patient or wrong anatomical site. The nurse must ensure that all universal protocol activities are documented and stored in the patient's medical record according to facility policy.

The universal protocol has three main components. First, a patient identification verification process must occur preoperatively. The patient must be correctly identified with two identifiers, such as name and date of birth. The nurse must ensure that the patient is able to confirm their identification verbally. If the patient is not conscious, other methods must be used to confirm identity, such as the medical record number. Other verification items include completed laboratory and diagnostic tests, blood products, implants, and special equipment that will be needed for the procedure.

Second, the surgical site must be marked prior to starting the procedure. The surgeon who will be present during the procedure must identify the anatomical location and physically mark the skin with a tool that is consistently used throughout the facility. The marking tool must be able to withstand skin preparation and draping.

The last component of the universal protocol is the time-out procedure. The time-out is performed immediately before the procedure is to begin. All healthcare providers involved in the surgery must be present for the time-out, such as the surgeon, circulating nurse, anesthesiologist, and operating room technician. The time-out ensures that everyone agrees with the procedure to be performed, confirms the identity of the patient, and verifies the correct surgical site. If a patient will be having multiple procedures during the surgery, a time-out must be performed before making each designated incision.

Anticipating the Need for Intraoperative Blood Transfusion/Salvage

The potential need for a blood transfusion during surgery must be assessed in the preoperative phase of surgery. In collaboration with the healthcare provider, the nurse must review laboratory results and identify medical conditions that may necessitate a blood transfusion. Some medical conditions to screen the patient for include anemias, blood clotting disorders, and medications that may increase the risk for bleeding such as anticoagulants or antiplatelet medications. Laboratory results that indicate a low platelet count, low hemoglobin, or a prolonged bleeding time should also be taken into consideration.

The nurse must also anticipate a blood transfusion for specific surgeries that may result in significant blood loss, such as trauma surgeries. Ruptured organs, compound fractures, and traumatic tissue injuries can all result in excessive blood loss intraoperatively. The nurse must ensure that the patient has preoperative laboratory work drawn to facilitate a blood transfusion. Blood typing and crossmatching are required to safely identify the patient's blood type and donor compatibility.

As part of the health history, nurses must identify any contraindications to blood transfusions. Patients may refuse blood products due to religious and cultural beliefs. Any surgical patient that is identified as having a contraindication must be given alternative options.

When a patient is identified as a risk for significant blood loss or when prevention of exposure to allogeneic blood is preferred, a blood salvage may be ordered. A blood salvage, also known as autotransfusion, reinfuses the patient's own blood after it is processed (separated, washed, and concentrated) intraoperatively. Blood salvage may also occur postoperatively. Postoperative blood salvage is most commonly ordered for major orthopedic surgeries, such as joint replacements. The blood is collected in a specialized surgical drain that is designed for performing an autologous blood transfusion. As with any blood transfusion, the nurse must be cautious to observe for any signs of fluid overload, infection, and emboli.

Proper Body Mechanics

Ergonomics is the science of matching the physical requirements of a job to the physical abilities of the worker. Musculoskeletal injuries can occur if physical demands are greater than the employee's physical capabilities. Body mechanics refers to how the body moves during activities of daily living. Understanding and practicing the use of proper body mechanics is imperative to preventing associate injury. The physical requirements of a job are explained during the interview process, and the physical capabilities of the associate are assessed during the pre-employment physical examination. Education on the use of proper body mechanics begins in nursing school and continues during employment. New associate orientation should include validation of proper body mechanics.

The perioperative environment can present potential hazards that increase risk of injury to the nurse. Examples of these are transferring the patient from the cart to the operating room bed, positioning the patient, and standing for prolonged periods. Repetitive motions, such as turning the head to one side for visualization of monitoring equipment and holding a retractor for an extended time period, can also present ergonomic hazards. Proper body mechanics should be consistently followed to prevent injury. There are three foundational principles of proper body mechanics that should be followed by perioperative nurses. First, bending at the hips and knees instead of at the waist uses the large muscle groups of the legs instead of the back muscles, and helps to prevent back injury. Second, standing with feet at about shoulder-width apart helps to reduce risk of injury by providing foundational support. Finally, the perioperative nurse should keep the back, neck, pelvis, and feet aligned when turning or moving. Twisting and bending at the neck and waist can increase risk of associate injury.

As a standard of care, many healthcare institutions have mandated use of **safe patient mobilization (SPM)** equipment in an effort to reduce associate injuries, as well as to promote patient safety. SPM equipment in the perioperative environment can be used during patient transfers and positioning.

Slide sheets are often used in patient transfers. These sheets are placed underneath the patient prior to lateral or vertical transfer. They decrease the surface tension, making transfers easier for the associates. However, since the slide sheets do decrease surface tension, they must be removed after use, so that the patient is not at risk of sliding off the operating room bed.

Inflatable blankets can be placed under the patient to assist in lateral transfers, as well. When engaged, the forced air blanket helps to support the weight of the patient, making lateral transfers easier. The mattress should be deflated after completion of transfer.

Another type of SPM equipment for perioperative use is lift equipment. Lift equipment works by placing a sling under the patient's limb or underneath the entire patient, connecting the sling to the lift machine, and programming the machine to lift the body to the desired height. The weight limits of these machines vary, so the perioperative nurse must ensure the patient's weight does not exceed the weight limit set by the manufacturer.

Proper Patient Positioning

The goal of **patient positioning** is to maintain patient comfort and safety while providing necessary exposure for the surgeon. The perioperative nurse, anesthesiologist, and surgeon work together in positioning the patient for surgery. During the preoperative interview, the patient should be asked questions regarding mobility limitations and restrictions. If mobility limitations exist, they should be considered when positioning the patient. For example, extreme pain and/or musculoskeletal injury can result if the patient with limited shoulder range of motion is positioned in a way that extends the shoulder past its range of motion.

Braden Scale

The **Braden Scale** is used to assess the risk of patients developing pressure ulcers (commonly known as bedsores). A pressure ulcer refers to internal and/or external damage that can occur in areas of the body where areas of bone are poorly cushioned by soft or adipose tissue (such as the tailbone). This is normally the result of low mobility in a patient, resulting in constant pressure placed on the bony area and therefore resulting in bruising of or breakage in the corresponding soft tissue, blood vessels, or skin.

The Braden Scale takes into account patients' sensory perception (whether they can feel areas of pressure), moisture (how damp an area is), activity (how much patients are able to generally move on their own or with assistance), mobility (how well patients are able to generally move on their own or with assistance), nutrition (patient intake of macronutrients, vitamins, and minerals that support bodily functions), and friction (if any areas are exposed to repeated rubbing or chafing). Based on this scale, patients will be categorized as at risk, moderate risk, high risk, or very high risk of developing a pressure ulcer. Nurse monitoring and patient care should be tailored to the patient's risk category.

Fowler

The **Fowler's Position** is a supine position that refers to placing patients in a supported (yet semi-reclined posture) of 45 to 60 degrees. This position takes the effort away from sitting up fully upright, but allows patient airways to open, necessary drainage to occur, and ease in eating and talking. The Fowler's Position can also take low, semi-, and high positioning. Low Fowler's position places the patient at a 15-degree inclination and is normally the positioning for a standard hospital bed. Semi-Fowler's positioning places the patient at an inclination of 35 to 40 degrees and is most commonly used for those who need feeding assistance. High Fowler's position is a normal seated position and best for patients that are recovering well, have strength, and can eat, drink, and breathe autonomously.

Nerve Injury

Nerve injury refers to damage of neurons that control autonomic, motor, and sensory processes in the body. These can range from mild (sometimes showing no symptoms) to severe (such as paralysis). Nerve injury can occur from chronic disease, traumatic injury, tight muscles, poor nutrition, or the presence of foreign bodies. Symptoms of nerve injury include tingling, pain, burning, weakness, partial or complete loss of sensory functions. Depending on the severity, these symptoms can be mild, intermittent, or debilitating. Severe nerve injuries, such as cauda equine syndrome, can cause organs to stop functioning.

Skin Integrity

Skin integrity refers to the health of a patient's skin. Skin with high integrity is free of open wounds, moist, and free of infection. This is an important factor in patient health as the skin is the largest barrier between external harmful agents and internal organs, bones, and tissues. When skin integrity is low, patients become more susceptible to infection, therefore reducing recovery time and quality of care while increasing poor health outcomes (including death). When providing care to patients, nurses should ensure that surgical and recovery positioning does not compromise the skin (i.e., leaving patients in a way that would make them prone to pressure ulcers). If patients already have compromised areas, medical staff should ensure that all precautions are made to keep the wound clean, bandaged, and free of pressure or friction.

Trendelenburg Position

The **Trendelenburg position** is a supine position in which the feet are elevated 15 to 30 degrees higher than the heart and head. It is most commonly utilized for patients who require pelvic or abdominal surgery; in a standard supine position, pelvic and abdominal organs are difficult to access due to the large and small intestines. The reverse Trendelenburg position is a supine position in which the head is elevated 15 to 30 degrees and the lower half of the body is angled toward the ground (rather than supine, such as in a Fowler's position). This position is most commonly used in patients who are at risk of pulmonary embolisms, asphyxiation, are having a procedure in the head or neck regions, or are overweight. The goal of reverse Trendelenburg positioning is to reduce pressure in the blood vessels of the head and neck.

Trendelenburg Position

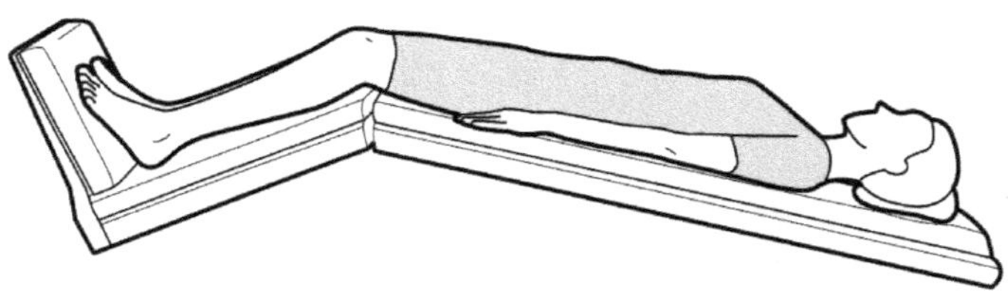

Reverse Trendelenburg Position

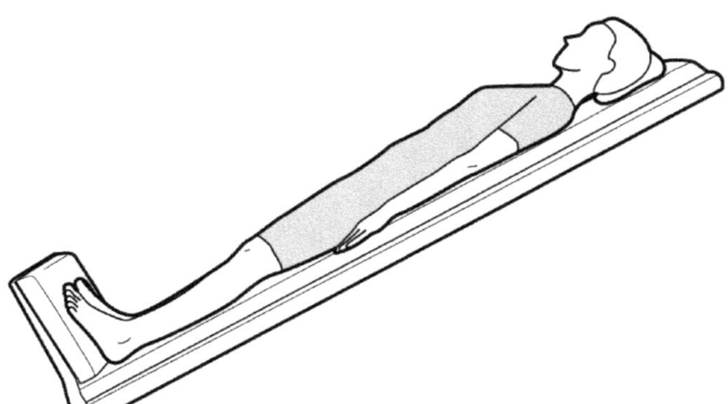

Patient Comorbidities

Patient **comorbidities** are also a consideration for positioning. If the patient has orthopnea (shortness of breath while lying flat), the patient should be positioned upright while awake. Morbidly obese patients often have orthopnea, in addition to being difficult to mechanically ventilate while under anesthesia. The anesthesiologist may need to elevate the head during surgery in order to promote effective ventilation. Conversely, the patient with hypotension may not tolerate sitting up. This patient may need to remain lying flat, or even with head down and legs elevated (Trendelenburg position).

Supine, Prone, and Lateral

There are three main positions used in surgery: supine, prone, and lateral. Variations of each of these three positions are also used. In supine, or dorsal recumbent, position, the patient lies on their back with legs on the bed. Patients undergoing most abdominal, open heart, and lower extremity procedures are in the supine position. In the supine position, the arms may be tucked at each side or placed on padded arm boards at each side. When tucking the arms, the health care provider should ensure that each of the patient's arm is placed snugly against the torso with the thumb facing upward.

Each elbow should be padded prior to tucking to protect the ulnar nerve. A pillow may be placed under the knees to alleviate pressure to the lower back. In addition to padding for the arms, a padded head rest is used to protect the head from pressure injury. To protect the heels from pressure injury, either a pillow or foam padding is placed behind the ankles to float the heels off of the bed. One variation of the supine position is lithotomy position. In lithotomy, the patient is supine with legs elevated in stirrups. This position is used for gynecological, urology, and colorectal procedures.

In prone position, the patient is placed abdominal-side down on the bed. This transition occurs after induction of anesthesia and placement of invasive monitoring lines. After the patient is transitioned from supine to prone position, the head is placed upon a padded head rest that supports the head and neck and allows room for the endotracheal tube and airway support. The patient's arms are bent at the elbows and placed at each side on padded arm rests. Pillows are placed under the knees and under the calves and feet for support. One variation of the prone position is the jackknife, or Kraske, position. In this variation, the patient is prone, and the bed is bent at the hip level to place the legs downward. Prone position may be used in back procedures and lower extremity vascular procedures.

Lateral positioning is used for chest, shoulder or arm, or lateral leg procedures, as well as some cardiac procedures. When the patient is in right lateral position, the patient is lying on the right side with the left side up. In this position, the right leg is bent to keep the hip at ninety degrees and the knee bent at about forty-five degrees. The top leg is relatively straight, and pillows are placed between the legs to provide support and padding. The upper extremity is placed across the chest and may be supported by pillows, a padded splint that is mounted to the bed, or another type of padded arm holder. The lower arm is supported with a pillow or padding and is placed on an arm board. The axillary area that is down on the bed is supported with an axillary roll. This roll alleviates pressure on the brachial plexus nerves. The patient is secured in position with either a beanbag mattress or lateral positioning rolls placed on front and back sides. These can be blanket rolls or gel rolls.

Regardless of the type of position, the patient is monitored for bony prominences and padding is used to protect them. The surgical patient is at risk for skin breakdown, especially in lengthy procedures.

Conflict Management

Conflict with Patients or Family Members

Nurses sometimes must contend with aggressive and violent behavior from patients or their family members who may be distressed. An aggressive or violent patient can be characterized by the exhibition of any nonverbal behaviors or verbal communication that intend to cause conflict, harm, pain, or injury. An aggressive or violent patient may invade personal space, make verbal threats or obscene gestures, mimic or follow through with physical threats, speak unnecessarily loudly or in a hostile manner, or be generally abusive in some other verbal or physical way. The causes motivating these behaviors are variable. Patients may show aggressive or violent behavior due to a psychiatric or physiological issue, such as drug abuse, delusions, head injuries, and infections of the brain. However, aggressive or violent behavior can also be a result of the patient's personal background and history, such as family upbringing, socioeconomic status, and current personal stressors.

Nurses should assess each patient for potential aggressive or violent behavior. This can include looking for known risk factors on intake forms (i.e., medical and psychological history, documented history of violence or substance abuse, history of detention or imprisonment, or personal stressors such as unemployment). This can also include assessing the patient directly and taking note of appearance, mental and physical state, pupil size, level of perspiration, mood, tone of speaking, and any comments made by the patient that could indicate current feelings of hostility or anger.

Nurses should be knowledgeable of their health care setting's policies and local laws as they relate to managing or sedating aggressive or violent patients. To protect the safety of medical personnel, the patient, and other patients in the vicinity, if a patient becomes visibly aggressive or violent, physical restraint may need to be provided by a dynamic team from the facility. In some cases, it may be necessary to administer antipsychotic medication or sedation.

Nurses should keep the following principles in mind when handling conflict or communicating with family members:

1. Recognize that the family is the constant in the patient's life while the service systems and personnel within those systems fluctuate

2. Be aware of family strengths and individuality and having respect for different methods of coping

3. Encourage and facilitating family-to-family support and networking

4. Share complete and unbiased information about the patient's care with family members on a continuing basis in a supportive manner

5. Design accessible healthcare delivery systems that are flexible, culturally competent, and responsive to family needs

Conflict and Collaboration Within the Perioperative Team

Common barriers to effective collaboration include conflicting professional opinions, ineffective communication related to the conflict, and incomplete assessment of the required elements of the care plan. Research indicates that physicians tend to stress cure-related activities while nurses tend to encourage care-related activities. This means that some resolution of these differences is required for effective communication. While collaboration is a necessary part of the process that matches the patient needs with the appropriate nursing competencies, it is also possible that the end product may be the best solution for the patient and at the same time be totally unacceptable to the patient. Collaborative team members should also be aware that while successful collaboration improves patient outcomes, research indicates that genuine collaborative efforts are rarely noted in patient care, often because the group is unable to integrate the diverse mental models of the group members.

Wound Classifications

The length and direction of the surgical incision affect wound healing for a few reasons. First, the longer the surgical incision, the more inflammation will be present due to the healing process. Second, the direction of the surgical incision influences the amount of pressure present at the surgical wound area. For example, a transverse (or horizontal) abdominal incision is preferred over a vertical abdominal incision because the transverse incision will result in less pressure placed upon it by the body, in comparison to a vertical incision. Stress on the incision impedes the ability of the body to properly heal.

Hemostasis is the absence of surgical bleeding, or cessation of the flow of blood. The sooner hemostasis is achieved, the sooner wound closure can occur, and the wound healing process can begin. Attempting to close the surgical wound in the absence of hemostasis contributes to moisture of the wound. Moisture in the wound area impedes the wound healing process.

If necrotic, or dead, tissue is present in the surgical wound, it must be removed or debrided to allow the body's wound healing process to take place. The surgeon chooses wound closure material based upon the type of surgery performed and individual patient characteristics, such as history of intolerance to suture material. For example, if the patient previously had an issue with wound healing after surgical closure with Vicryl suture, the surgeon may choose to use PDS suture this time.

Surgical Wound Classification Decision Tree

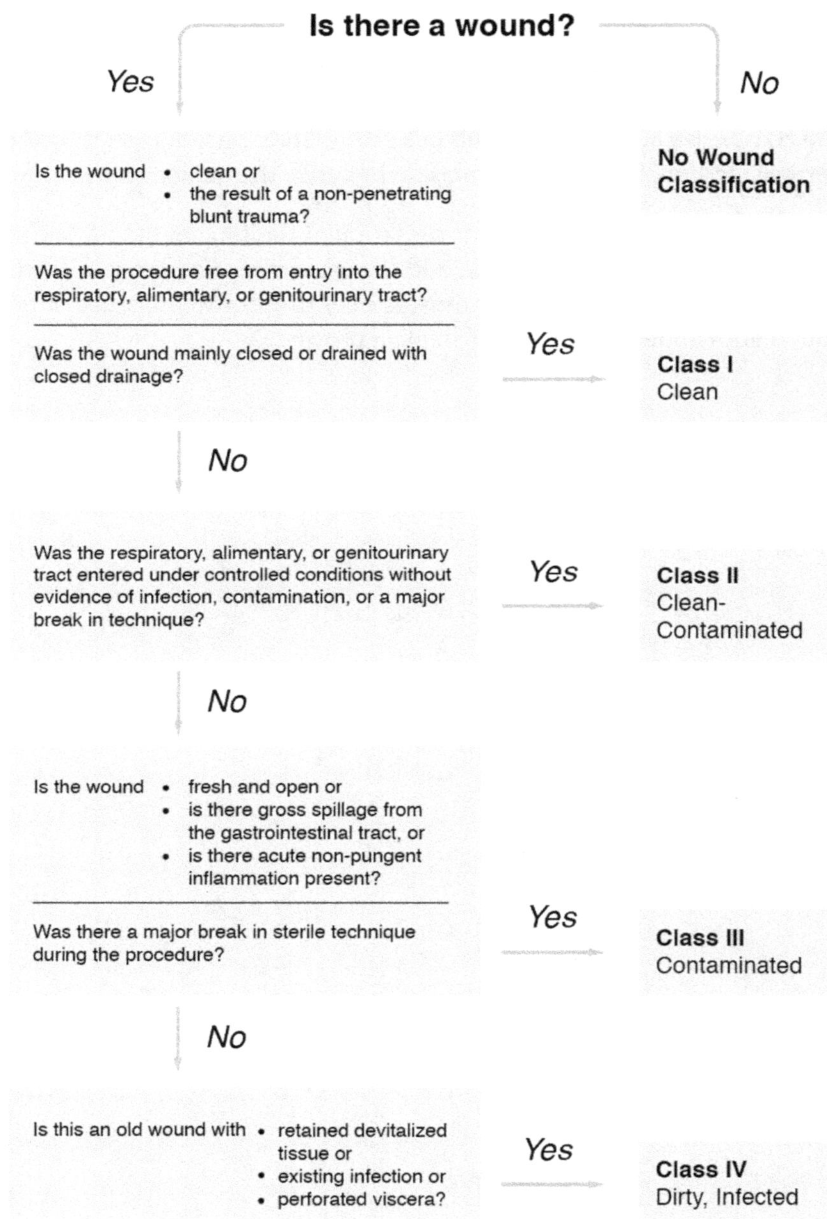

A **surgical wound** is classified according to the level of contamination at the time of surgery. Classifying the surgical wound is one way to predict postoperative risk of SSI. The Centers for Disease Control and Prevention (CDC) guidelines for prevention of surgical site infection, released in 1999, identify four categories of surgical wounds: Class I (clean), Class II (clean contaminated), Class III (contaminated), and Class IV (dirty or infected). In Class I, no breaks in sterile technique are encountered in the perioperative encounter. The respiratory, genital, alimentary, or infected urinary tracts are not entered.

A Class I wound is primarily closed, and no open drains are used (such as Penrose and Jackson-Pratt drains). Examples of clean surgical wounds are sternotomy, mastectomy, and leg revascularization incisions.

A Class II surgical wound is one that involves the respiratory, alimentary, genital, or urinary tracts under normal circumstances. No obvious contamination is present, and no breaks in sterile technique are encountered. Surgeries resulting in clean contaminated surgical wounds are hysterectomy, tracheostomy, lobectomy of the lung, appendectomy, prostatectomy, and colon resection.

A Class III surgical wound is encountered in a surgical procedure with a major break in sterile technique, spillage from the gastrointestinal tract, or open, accidental wounds. Incisions with acute inflammation also fall into Class III. Examples of Class III surgical wounds are open fractures, penetrating wounds, emergent sternotomy with cardiac massage, and surgeries performed using unsterile instruments.

The Class IV surgical wound involves existing clinical infection, perforated viscera, visible purulent material, or an old traumatic wound with necrotic tissue. Class IV indicates microorganisms that can cause postoperative SSI are present before the time of surgery.

Accurate identification of surgical wound class is important in predicting the patient's risk for SSI. Ultimately, the surgeon determines the surgical wound class. The surgeon may also use the surgical wound classification system in determining the appropriate preoperative antibiotic prophylaxis.

Wound Healing

Wound healing occurs in stages from the immediate postoperative period, lasting up to a few years after surgery. The perioperative nurse should understand the factors that affect wound healing and identify opportunities for patient education to promote proper wound healing and decrease risk of SSI. Patient conditions that may adversely influence the body's wound healing capability are malnutrition, hyperglycemia, obesity, smoking, and respiratory compromise. These conditions contribute to lack of blood and nutrient supply to tissue, therefore decreasing wound healing capability.

There are three stages in wound healing: inflammation, proliferation, and remodeling. The inflammation phase begins in the immediate postoperative period and lasts about six days. During the inflammation phase, hemostasis occurs. After hemostasis, phagocytosis takes place. In phagocytosis, the white blood cells "clean up" the area by eliminating foreign particles. **Edema** also occurs in the inflammation phase. Edema, or swelling at the surgical site, is a result of the immunological system signaling blood flow to the area to promote wound healing. Proliferation occurs around one to two days postoperatively and continues for approximately three weeks. During proliferation, the wound tissue appears reddened; this is from the formation of granulation tissue. Blood vessels of surrounding tissue are replenished, and scab formation begins. The final phase of wound healing is the remodeling phase. The remodeling phase begins at about three weeks after surgery and can last for two years postoperatively. During remodeling, collagen fibers connect together, and scar tissue eventually forms.

There are three methods for facilitating wound healing. These are primary union, granulation, and delayed primary closure. Each of these three methods involves inflammation, proliferation, and remodeling, to some degree. Primary union happens in surgical cases with aseptically made wounds with little or no tissue damage. Primary union occurs in ideal surgical conditions, and it is the preferred method for wound healing. Granulation is the second way wound healing may be achieved. The wound is left open and heals from the inside out. Infected wounds are often left open after debridement for granulation to occur. Delayed primary closure is used in contaminated or traumatic cases with a high risk of infection. The wound is typically packed with gauze and monitored for infection and drainage. On postoperative day three to five, the wound is closed. Delayed primary closure may be used in cases of compartment syndrome, where swelling is highly anticipated.

Intraoperative factors that influence the wound healing process are sterile technique, length and direction of incision, hemostasis, wound moisture, presence of necrotic tissue, the material used to close the surgical wound, tension applied by the surgeon in wound closure, and stress on the wound after surgery. When the perioperative team uses proper sterile technique, the chance for microorganisms to enter the surgical wound is decreased. Keeping the surgical wound free of these microorganisms helps to promote proper wound healing.

Maintaining Wound Dressings

Incisions created during surgery increase the patient's risk of infection. Postoperatively, the nurse will manage various wound dressings and products that prevent contamination of the wound. The type of dressing is dependent on the location, size, and depth of the wound or surgical incision. Regardless of the type of dressing, the nurse must look for signs of bleeding, dehiscence, and evisceration postoperatively. Any indication of hemorrhage or wound complications should be reported to the healthcare provider or surgeon immediately. The nurse must also ensure that patients are premedicated with analgesics prior to performing a dressing change to ensure adequate pain management.

Laparoscopic surgeries are minimally invasive. The incisions are typically small and do not require staples or sutures to keep them approximated. The types of wound dressings used for these incisions are transparent films or adhesives to allow for visualization of the incision. Hydrocolloid dressings are occlusive or semi-occlusive and prevent wound contamination. However, these dressings are not absorbent and are typically used for wounds with light drainage.

Foam dressings covered with hydrophilic polyurethane film are used for surgical wounds that are expected to produce light to heavy amounts of drainage. These dressings can remain in place for 3 to 7 days, depending on the amount of exudate. Skin graft surgeries will be covered with antimicrobial dressings or collagens to protect and prevent infection to the graft or donor site.

Complex surgical wounds or wounds that become complicated postoperatively may have negative pressure wound therapy applied. Negative pressure therapy provides high absorbency of drainage, decreases bacterial colonization, and stimulates the formation of granulation tissue. Negative wound therapy requires a sponge over the incision that must be exchanged every 2 to 3 days depending on the amount of exudate collected.

Management of Intraoperative Activities

Room Preparation

Prior to the day of surgery, the staff should review the upcoming cases to prepare for any consignment items or specialty items. In some cases, vendors may be required to bring these items to the OR for processing the day before the scheduled procedure. If the staff is not proactive, the case may be delayed or canceled on the day of surgery, which is detrimental both to the facility and the patient.

When preparing for a case, the circulator should review the required equipment, supplies, and personnel and ensure availability. For example, specialized equipment may be required in multiple scheduled cases, and the circulator should verify that the equipment will be available when needed before starting the procedure.

Equipment and Supplies

Surgical instruments are categorized by their purpose. Generally, instruments fall into three categories: cutting instruments, clamps, and graspers/holders. Cutting instruments are those used for cutting tissue. Knife handles are used for holding the surgical blade. The surgical blade may be used to make skin incision, to incise or puncture a blood vessel, or to dissect a portion of tissue. To decrease the chance of sharps injury to the surgical team members, surgical blades with built-in safety devices should be used. The safety device is designed to cover the sharp while the blade is passed between the surgical team members. Two types of scissors are used in surgery: tissue and suture scissors. Tissue scissors are used for cutting tissue. Metzenbaum and Mayo are two types of tissue scissors. Suture scissors are used to cut sutures and other surgical supplies, such as paper and synthetic graft material. Bandage scissors and wire cutters are examples of suture scissors. Scissors are also used after skin incision to dissect tissue for exposure to the surgical area.

Clamps are used to hold areas together. The type of clamp used depends on the amount and type of tissue to be clamped together. Some clamps provide total occlusion, while others are used for partial occlusion of an area. A clamp has "teeth" that come together when the clamp is engaged. The teeth may be fine or robust, depending on the type of tissue the clamp is meant for. A commonly used surgical clamp is the hemostat. The hemostat is used to minimize blood loss by clamping vessels together. Hemostats come in a variety of sizes and may be straight or curved.

Graspers and holders are another category of instruments. They are designed to hold or grasp tissue and provide traction away from the surgical area. Graspers come in a multitude of styles and are selected by the surgeon depending on the type and amount of tissue to be grasped. There are tissue holders as well as needle holders, or needle drivers.

Other surgical instruments include staplers, forceps, saws, scopes, and retractors. Staplers are used to wedge away organ tissue, such as lung tissue for biopsy. They are also used for stapling the skin closed at the end of the procedure. Forceps are used to pick up tissue. Saws can be used for sternotomy or cutting away bone in orthopedic procedures. Scopes are used for visualization in minimally invasive procedures such as laparoscopy and thoracoscopy. Retractors are used to separate tissue and provide visualization for the surgical area. Retractors come in a variety of sizes and may be used for retracting a small blood vessel or for retracting something as large as an entire abdomen.

In addition to surgical instruments, other supplies are needed to successfully perform a surgical procedure. Sutures are used to sew vessels together and to close the skin layers at the end of the procedure. Sponges, such as laparotomy and gauze, are used to absorb blood away from the surgical area. Sponges used in the surgical field have x-ray detectable material in them so they can be visualized on x-ray in the event of an incorrect surgical sponge count at the end of the case. Disposable knife blades are attached to knife handle instruments for making skin incision or for incising vascular tissue. Surgical drapes are applied after skin prep is completed to maintain the sterile field integrity. Surgical gowns and gloves are worn by all members of the sterile field. Surgical implants are used in certain procedures, including aortic valve replacement, permanent pacemaker insertion, and lower extremity bypass graft. Surgical dressings are applied at the end of the procedure to protect the surgical area and minimize risk for surgical site infection.

Examples of anesthesia supplies are syringes, intravenous catheter access needles, intravenous tubing sets, ventilator circuits, endotracheal tubes, ambu bags, tongue depressors, alcohol pads, and tape.

Surgical equipment is used, along with surgical instruments and supplies, to perform the surgical procedure. Some equipment is standard for all surgical cases, while others are used for specific cases only. As technology changes and grows, new and different types of equipment are introduced into the perioperative environment. Robotic surgery, for example, has become very popular and requires a specific set of equipment.

In general, each operating room is equipped with the following: a monitor for patient vital signs, a surgical bed, a fire extinguisher, gas supply ports, vacuum ports for suction, suction canisters, an electrosurgical cautery machine, stools, tables for workspace and supplies, and extra tables for sterile set-up. Most surgical procedures require an anesthesia machine that is equipped with ETCO2 monitoring and a ventilator circuit. Some operating rooms contain a defibrillator, while others have a central location for the defibrillator and other emergency equipment. A monitoring tower, which includes gas supply, camera source, and light source, is used in minimally invasive cases for visualization. A pneumatic tourniquet is used in vascular and orthopedic procedures to reduce blood flow at the surgical site during critical points of the operation. X-ray equipment may be indicated to provide radiology imaging intraoperatively. A surgical laser is used in select cases for tissue ablation.

Packaging and Sterilization

Packaging has a shelf life or duration in which a pack has a "sterile" status. This time frame not only pertains to how long an item can stay on the shelf while retaining its sterility, but also has an "event-related" component under which a product remains sterile until the occurrence of various events that breach sterility. For example, products that are dropped on the floor, torn open, or get wet are no longer sterile, even if they have not met their designated sterility expiration date. There are many protocols for sterile packages that are in place to sustain the life of the pack.

There should be no contact with the sterile packs upon removal from the sterilizing system for up to sixty minutes. Bacteria may form if a freshly sterilized pack is placed on a cool surface without being given time to cool down. As a result, condensation forms on the package and makes it vulnerable to bacteria that can easily penetrate the package and multiply, thus making the package unsterile.

Perioperative personnel must store sterile packs in locations that are clean and dry, only handling packages when necessary. The environment should be temperature-controlled and have low humidity and good ventilation. The storage place for these materials should be a location with limited access.

Open shelves should not be a storage location of choice, but rather a space with cabinets that close. If there is any utilization of open shelves for storage of these packs, there should be space between the ceiling and the floor. The rack closest to the ceiling should be no closer than eighteen inches, and the lowest shelf should not be closer than eight to ten inches to the floor. Also, packs should not reside on shelves that touch the walls. These dimensions allow for the best ventilation and reduce the risk of moisture accumulation on any of the packs.

Dynamic Air Removal and Gravity Displacement

Dynamic air removal and gravity displacement are two methods of steam sterilization that are used to disinfect medical devices. In a dynamic air removal system, instruments that need sterilization are placed in a holding bag which is then placed into a chamber. As steam forcefully enters the chamber, the air that was previously in the chamber is actively removed through a vacuum mechanism. This clears the chamber and allows steam to enter the holding bag and sterilize the instruments. The vacuum mechanism is then used to remove the steam and dry the instruments.

Gravity displacement sterilization uses the force of gravity, rather than an attached vacuum, to remove the air that was previously in the chamber out. As long as the steam is at a hotter temperature than the air in the chamber, the pressure difference will push the air out. The dynamic air removal process allows sterilization to occur in under five minutes, whereas the gravity displacement process can take about half an hour. When sterilization is complete, the instruments should be left in the chamber until cool and all moisture has evaporated. Touching the instruments before all moisture has evaporated will likely lead to contamination. In gravity displacement systems, complete drying can take two hours or more.

Cost Containment and Product Evaluation

There is a lot of specialized equipment and types of materials used in the OR, and many of these items are rather costly. And while the overall costs have generally increased, many facilities are being reimbursed less for procedures. In order to react to this, many facilities have looked toward material costs and material wastage to reduce their operating costs. While the circulator may not be directly responsible for the financial success of the department, they should participate in efforts to improve the facility's operational and financial success.

One area of concentration has been on branded vs. nonbranded items. This struggle is very similar to what was seen in pharmaceuticals with brand vs. generic drugs. Frequently, the vendor representative for a branded material, piece of equipment, or drug may introduce their product, which may be more expensive than a similar nonbranded product. Prior to moving forward with stocking this branded product, OR management should review for similar, less expensive options. This also may require the cooperation of surgeons, who may have a personal preference for the more expensive option.

Another consideration is single-use items vs. items that can be reprocessed. While many believe single-use items pose less risk of infection or contamination, reprocessed items that are sterilized correctly may be a less expensive option for some types of materials. For example, many surgeons prefer disposable trocars, but there are stainless steel trocars that can be reprocessed for multiple uses that may reduce the operating costs to the facility. This again requires buy-in from the surgeon, which is why the entire multidisciplinary team should be involved in cost-containment or cost-reduction initiatives.

Another area of cost containment involves personnel costs. Staffing is typically the highest operating cost of the OR, followed by expenditures on materials and inventory. When managing the staff of an OR, the nurse should ensure that staff members are not unnecessarily working overtime.

Product Evaluation and Selection

When products and materials are being evaluated and selected, the circulator should participate as needed. In most cases, the surgeon will have the majority of the input, followed by the OR manager, who must consider the surgeon's preference in relation to the relative cost of the item. Frequently, the vendor representative will be present during product evaluation and selection, and the circulator should pay attention to any specific instructions about preparing or using the product.

Cost-Containment Measures

As facilities are asked to do more with fewer supplies, the staff should always cooperate with cost-containment measures. Management should constantly review product alternatives in the market to ensure they are ordering and using the most cost-effective items. One key component of cost containment is surgeon engagement. Many surgeons have grown accustomed to OR management accommodating their personal preference items, regardless of cost. However, recent efforts have included involving surgeons in reviewing their case costs compared to their peers and material costs of their personal preferences compared to less expensive replacement items. In most cases, when the surgeons are made aware of their impact to the overall case cost, they are willing to compromise for comparable equipment and materials.

The circulator should also be aware of items that may be more expensive and not always required for a procedure. If there are materials that are infrequently used and the item is expensive, the circulator should discuss with the team and determine which materials should be opened to prepare for the case and what items may be held in availability to open as needed. This helps ensure that materials are not wasted unnecessarily.

Coordinate Preventive Maintenance on Equipment

At most facilities, the biomedical engineering staff will be responsible for coordinating and performing maintenance on equipment. However, because some of the equipment will be in short supply at the facility, the circulator may be directly impacted by a single piece of equipment being unavailable. For equipment requiring preventive maintenance, the circulator should assist as needed. If there is anticipated maintenance, the OR director should cross-reference the OR schedule to determine if there is an ideal time to perform this maintenance or proactively check to see what cases may be impacted by this loss of equipment. In some cases, it may be possible to have another facility loan needed equipment. However, this typically requires advanced notice, so the team should attempt to coordinate as much as possible in advance.

Maintenance and tracking of robotics equipment are of particular importance. At many facilities, there may be only one robot and a very limited supply of instruments. When the case is complete, typically the robot will display how many uses are left for the instrument. The circulator should ensure that there is an adequate supply of replacement instruments so that future cases are not impacted by lacking equipment.

Educating Health Care Team Members

The circulator plays a key role in supervising other health care members. The circulator should be constantly aware of personnel entering and exiting the OR. Every additional person in the OR increases the risk of contamination or infection, so visitors should be minimized when possible. The circulator should always use their judgment when asked to accommodate visitors or students. At some facilities, certain procedures, such as joint replacement surgery, may have restrictions on visitors or students because these cases pose the highest risk for poor outcomes if there is contamination. The circulator should comply with the facility policy and, as the patient advocate, ensure that other health care team members are providing the safest environment

Every circulator remembers their first day in the OR and should appreciate the importance of education and mentorship. The environment in the OR is unique, and many nursing programs do not offer OR training. For that reason, many nursing students or new graduates in the OR may have little to no education on OR etiquette or expected behavior. While the patient's safety should be the highest priority, the circulator should also provide the appropriate attention and education to other health care members.

Experienced nurses working in the perioperative area have a duty to supervise and guide graduate nurses and registered nurses who are new to the nursing profession or the area of practice. Perioperative nursing incorporates several phases, and care must be taken to ensure nurses perform interventions within their scope of practice.

The preoperative phase includes obtaining a health history of the patient, reviewing laboratory and diagnostic results, and performing physical assessments to ensure the patient is stable for the procedure. Education is also an important aspect of preoperative nursing. The patient must know beforehand what the expectations of their recovery will be. The administration of medications preoperatively is a crucial step in preparing the patient for surgery. Supervisory nurses must ensure that staff nurses are knowledgeable about the medications they are administering, are aware of their indications, and are vigilant about possible adverse effects. As coordinators, nurses must ensure all members of the healthcare team are ready to perform the universal protocol before the start of the procedure.

In the intraoperative setting, circulating nurses have the responsibility to ensure that all members of the operative team are maintaining safe practices in the operating room. These practices include patient safety and infection control. Any unsafe practices, such as breaking sterile technique, incorrectly positioning a patient, or performing interventions that can cause patient harm should be addressed. Education should be provided for any member of the healthcare team that requires knowledge on safe practices.

In the postoperative setting, the nurse has the primary duty of monitoring the patient for complications and ensuring pain management. Any medications that are required to maintain stability of the patient's health must be ordered or included in the postoperative protocol. Supervisory nurses have a duty to ensure that staff nurses are administering medications as ordered. Due to the possibility of postoperative complications, any change in the patient's condition should immediately be reported to the surgeon or healthcare provider.

Personnel Delegation

When supervising and delegating responsibilities in the OR, the managing circulator should always be cognizant of team members' scope of practice. In order to provide a safe environment for the patient and to maintain integrity of the sterile field, tasks should only be assigned to personnel when it is within their scope of practice. The circulator should also take into account the urgency of the task with respect to the best interests of the patient. For example, if an item needs to be opened onto the sterile field prior to the procedure, the circulator may delegate this task to a student requiring supervision and instruction to ensure there is no contamination. However, during an emergency situation, the circulator may decide that it is not appropriate to delegate any tasks to personnel requiring additional assistance or supervision in order to meet the critical needs of the emergency situation.

Supervising Visitors

In addition to the regular members of the surgical team, the circulator should also be prepared for visitors in the OR, and these visitors may or may not be familiar with the importance of sterile technique, depending on their roles. One of the main priorities of the circulator when managing non-OR personnel is the integrity of the sterile field. Regardless of the level of experience, the circulator should ensure that only necessary personnel are present in the OR and kindly ask nonessential personnel to exit the room when appropriate.

Vendors are frequent visitors to the OR, especially in orthopedic surgery and neurosurgery. The role of the vendor in the OR is to educate the surgeon and staff on how their products should be used. Vendors are typically required to maintain certification with the Association of perioperative Registered Nurses (AORN) and other accrediting bodies, which includes knowledge of sterile technique and OR protocol. However, the circulator should always be aware of the risk to sterile technique. In addition, vendors should be aware of patient privacy and should not enter the OR until the patient is draped and also should exit prior to closure.

Medical and nursing students, along with allied health care students, may be present in the OR. The students will have varying levels of OR experience and should be monitored accordingly. Especially in pediatric procedures, family members may be invited into the OR to help ease the patient's anxiety during induction of anesthesia. Family members will likely have little to no experience in the OR and not be aware of the principles of sterile technique.

Supervise Non-OR Personnel

When a vendor arrives to the OR, the staff should ensure that they have followed the appropriate protocols to check in at the facility, which should include confirming their credentials are up to date. Some facilities also require vendors to wear a different color scrub hat to make it visibly apparent that they are not a staff member. During the procedure, the circulator should monitor the vendor to ensure the sterile field is not compromised, and as it is outside the scope of their responsibilities, the vendor should not open items onto the sterile field. Further, while the vendor and surgeon may have a personal relationship outside of the OR, the circulator should speak up if they feel the vendor is distracting the surgeon from the case.

Students should also be carefully monitored because, even if they have received training, their skills and awareness of the sterile field are likely undeveloped. When delegating tasks to students, the circulator should ensure they are qualified to perform these tasks and supervise as needed.

When escorting other visitors or family members into the sterile environment, the circulator should assume that they have no knowledge of sterile technique and supervise them appropriately. The circulator should also ensure they wear the proper PPE and provide instructions for donning this equipment. When these visitors are in the OR, they should be instructed to maintain a safe distance from any sterile tables or equipment. When the visitor or family member is no longer needed, the circulator should escort them out of the OR and provide instructions for removing PPE.

Managing Healthcare Industry Representative Presence in the OR

Every healthcare facility should have policies regarding the presence of a healthcare industry representative (HCIR) in the operating room. HCIRs are associated with manufacturers of medical devices and supplies, and they can provide knowledge, expertise, and technical assistance to the surgical team during the procedure. For example, a hospital has acquired a new negative pressure wound therapy device. Although training is required before its use, surgeons may not be familiar with best practices regarding the device. An HCIR would provide guidance within the operating room to ensure that the device is placed correctly and functioning properly before the procedure is completed.

Facility policies should include several elements to ensure that the patient's health, privacy, and confidentiality are maintained during the surgery. The presence of an HCIR in the operating room must be approved by the appropriate hospital authority. HCIRs should be screened for health concerns and provided with an orientation to the facility. Identification must be worn at all times to distinguish their role in the operating room. Due to the risk of infection during surgery, verification of the HCIR's education and training regarding aseptic and sterile technique must be performed.

Patients should also be informed of the HCIR's presence and purpose in the operating room during their procedure. Patients must provide consent before the procedure begins. It is important to note that the HCIR's primary role is an advisor. The nurse must ensure the HCIR does not perform activities outside of their scope. For example, an HCIR cannot be involved in medical decision making or have direct patient contact during the surgery.

Environmental Stewardship

"Going green" continues, even in the OR! Similar to goals of controlling costs, the circulator should be aware of any programs at the facility to encourage minimization of waste and recycling. For example, many facilities encourage staff to recycle certain types of single-use equipment, such as LigaSure scalpels. However, the circulator should be well informed of which pieces of equipment can be reprocessed and which pieces should be discarded. Also, some facilities may encourage discarding visibly clean, unused but opened items in designated bins that may be reprocessed for needy facilities, such as ORs in third-world countries.

Another program that contributes to a more sustainable environment is recycling clean plastic, cardboard, or foam wrapping and padding. When possible, this should be done prior to the patient entering the OR to ensure the recycled materials are clean.

Practice Quiz

1. Aside from the operating room, where might a surgical procedure be performed in the hospital setting?
    a. Oncology unit
    b. Critical care unit
    c. Radiology department
    d. Dialysis unit

2. Which of the following is a benefit associated with a minimally invasive surgical procedure?
    a. Intraoperative time is decreased
    b. Need for urinary catheterization is eliminated
    c. Risk for SSI is decreased
    d. Anesthetic gases are not used

3. The surgical time out is documented by which member of the surgical team?
    a. Perioperative nurse
    b. Anesthesiologist
    c. Surgeon
    d. Surgical technologist

4. The surgical procedure note is documented by the surgeon post-procedure. What piece of information is included in this documentation?
    a. Perioperative medication administration record
    b. Central line insertion note
    c. Tourniquet inflation and deflation times
    d. Estimated blood loss

5. Evidence-based guidelines support the use of what type of perioperative documentation system as a best practice?
    a. Carbon copied documentation files
    b. Binder kept on surgical unit
    c. Handwritten nursing care plans
    d. Electronic health record (EHR)

See answers on next page.

Answer Explanations

1. B: If the patient is critically ill and deemed too unstable for transport to the operating room, the surgeon may opt to perform the procedure at the bedside. The oncology unit is not considered a critical care area, so the patient on this unit would not be considered too unstable for transport. The radiology and dialysis areas are not inpatient units and would not accommodate a surgical procedure.

2. C: The risk of SSI is lower due to the smaller incisional area. Intraoperative time is not necessarily decreased; in fact, it may be longer. The need for urinary catheterization and anesthetic gases is not eliminated in minimally invasive procedures.

3. A: The perioperative nurse documents the surgery record, perioperative medication administration record, surgical time out, and nursing pathway. The surgical time out is not documented by the surgeon, anesthesiologist, or surgical technologist.

4. D: The surgical procedure note includes a description of the surgical steps in sequence, estimated blood loss, surgical specimens, and outcome of surgery. The perioperative medication administration record and tourniquet times are completed by the perioperative nurse. The central line insertion note is done by the anesthesiologist.

5. D: Evidence-based guidelines suggest the use of an electronic health record (EHR) as best practice. Carbon copied documentation and handwritten care plans are outdated and are not considered best practice. The use of binders on surgical units is not supported as a means of perioperative documentation.

Communication and Documentation

One skill that all perioperative nurses must possess is effective communication. Perioperative nurses will also have to engage various individuals throughout the different stages of a surgical procedure, including the patient, the patient's family, the surgeon, the anesthetist, and other members of the health care delivery team. Perioperative nurses must be able to execute effective listening skills, and they have to use the information provided to decipher what information poses to be of significant risk for the patient. Communication may be verbal or written; thus, the perioperative nurse should be able to review and process a lot of information as well as identify which pieces of data are most relevant and require further discussion.

Documentation

Clinical Documentation

Clinical documentation of each phase of the perioperative spectrum serves as a baseline of care coordination and communication while providing for patient safety. It provides a historical snapshot of care given to the patient and the patient's response to each intervention by various members of the health care team.

While most documentation is done electronically, nurses should also be familiar with the policies and procedures for paper documentation in the event of computer system downtime.

Intraoperative Report Content
Names of Professionals caring for patient/supporting care
Preoperative and postoperative diagnosis
Type of surgical procedure
Surgical sites
Specimens that were collected
Positioning
Medications
Electrosurgical unit and number
IV lines
Level of consciousness
Prosthesis
Skin prep

In an effort to adhere to federal and state regulations and accreditation protocol, many facilities maintain documentation of invasive or operative procedures. An intraoperative report is a permanent part of the patient's record, and it can provide insight into the patient's status postoperatively.

Pre-operative Record

Pre-operative

Patient Name .... Surgeon .... Date ....

Procedure ....

Arrival .... **ID** ☐ Verbal ☐ Nameband **Pt Verbalizes** ☐ Procedure Site ☐ Surgeon **NPO** Since ....

Allergies: ☐ NDA ☐ Latex ☐ Other .... ☐ Drugs ....

Lab Data: ☐ CBC ☐ Urinalysis ☐ Chemistry ☐ Coag Studies .... ☐ Pregnancy Test

Reports: ☐ EKG ☐ Chest ☐ H & P ☐ Other

Consents: ☐ Surgical ☐ Blood ☐ Anaesthesia

Blood Products - # of units in OR ....

Blood Bank .... ☐ Type and Screen .... ☐ Type and Cross ....

☐ Autologus .... ☐ Directed .... ☐ Homologus ....

Equipment: ☐ IV's ☐ Foley ☐ Ventilator ☐ Cardiac Monitor ☐ IABP ☐ Other ....

Prosthesis: ☐ None ☐ Ophthalmic ☐ Optic ☐ Dental ☐ Jewellery Disposition of Prosthesis ....

Orientation: ☐ Awake ☐ Oriented ☐ Sedated ☐ Confused ☐ Agitated ☐ Crying

Implants / Other Comments: ....

.... RN SIGNATURE ....

Intra-operative

Identification: ☐ Verbal ☐ Nameband Scrub Nurse: ☐ Sees Permits ☐ Aware of Allergies

Skin Condition: ☐ Intact ☐ Presence of Lesions - Type/Location ....

Skin Prep: ☐ Betadine ☐ Hibiclens ☐ Other ....

Position: ☐ Supine ☐ Prone ☐ Lithonomy ☐ Lateral ☐ Jackknife ☐ Fracture Table ☐ Other .... Positioned by ....

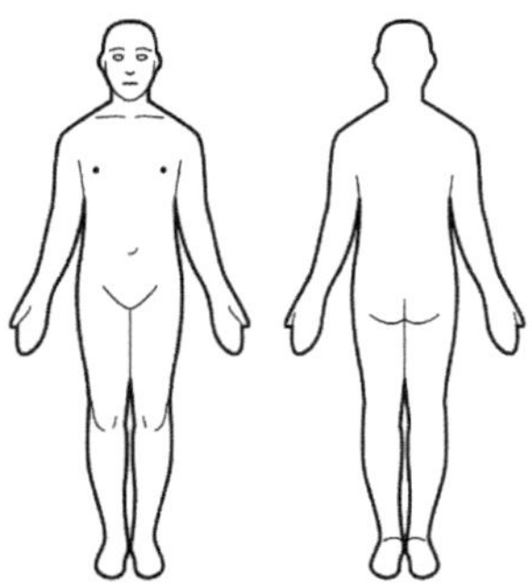

Equipment Codes:

= - Safety Strap applied by ....
X - Grounding Pad applied by ....
T - Tourniquet applied by ....
Δ - Pressure Pads applied by ....
S - Sandbag applied by ....
R - Roll applied by ....
A - Action Donut applied by ....
Z - Zoll Defib Pad applied by ....

Supports:

☐ Kidney Rest ....
☐ Stirrups ....
☐ Arms@Side ....
☐ Arms on Armboard ....
☐ Action Pads ....
☐ Black Leg Positioner ....
☐ Bean Bag ....

Tourniquet Unit # .... mm/Hg .... Inflated .... Deflated ....

Warning Blanket Unit # .... Temp .... On .... Off ....

Electrocautery Unit # .... Coag @ .... Cut @ ....

Pad # .... Exp. Date .... ESU Pad Skin Site ....

Defibrillator # .... Time / Joules ....

BiPolar Unit # .... Setting .... Other Equipment ....

Comments ....

.... RN SIGNATURE ....

Perioperative Checklists

Perioperative checklists are an excellent method to validate the execution of processes and procedures and are an essential pathway for communication among multiple disciplines. They enable health care professionals to adhere to standards and identify potential trends that may impact operational procedures, decrease adverse events, reduce medical errors, address unusual occurrences, and affect the overall quality of care. The arrangement of data on a checklist appears in a format that is easier for staff to process.

Some organizations have chosen to adopt the World Health Organization's (WHO's) Surgical Safety Checklist in an effort to increase patient safety while further enhancing documentation standards. The intent of this tool is to reduce the number of complications and poor outcomes that have an association with surgical procedures before, during, and after surgery.

Surgical Safety Checklist

Before induction of anaesthesia

with at least nurse and anaesthetist

Has the patient confirmed his/her identity, site, procedure, and consent?

- ☐ YES

Is the site marked?

- ☐ YES
- ☐ Not applicable

Is the anaesthesia machine and medication check complete?

- ☐ YES

Is the pulse oximeter on the patient and functioning?

- ☐ YES

Does patient have a:

Known allergy?

- ☐ NO
- ☐ YES

Difficult airway or aspiration risk?

- ☐ NO
- ☐ YES, and equipment/ assistance available

Risk of >500 ml blood loss (7 ml/kg in children)?

- ☐ NO
- ☐ YES, and two IVs/central access and fluids planned

Before skin incision

with nurse, anaesthetist and surgeon

- ☐ Confirm all team members have introduced themselves by name and role
- ☐ Confirm the patient's name, procedure, and where the incision will be made

Has antibiotic prophylaxis been given within the last 60 minutes?

- ☐ YES
- ☐ Not applicable

Anticipated Critical Events

To Surgeon:

- ☐ What are the critical or non-routine steps?
- ☐ How long will the case take?
- ☐ What is the anticipated blood loss?

To Anaesthetist:

- ☐ Are there any patient-specific concerns?

To Nursing Team:

- ☐ Has sterility (including indicator results) been confirmed?
- ☐ Are there equipment issues or any concerns?

Is essential imaging displayed?

- ☐ YES
- ☐ Not applicable

Before patient leaves operating room

with nurse, anaesthetist and surgeon

Nurse verbally confirm:

- ☐ The name of the procedure
- ☐ Completion of instrument, sponge and needle counts
- ☐ Specimen labelling (*read specimen labels aloud, including patient name*)
- ☐ Whether there are any equipment problems to be addressed

To Surgeon, Anaesthetist and Nurse:

- ☐ What are the key concerns for recovery and management of this patient?

However, it is important to note that, while studies show that checklists can be effective in standardizing practices, they are only effective if everyone from various disciplines commit to using them. Also, various professionals within each of these disciplines must respect the perspectives and expertise of one another.

Standardized Communication Tool

A standardized communication tool sets the same parameters for requested information each time an instance communication occurs. By asking for specific answers to the same set of questions, regardless of who is sending information and who is receiving it, standardized communication tools aim to reduce variability in communication, incomplete or partial communication, and irrelevant communication. In the medical setting, standardized communication tools are associated with improved quality of care, improved patient outcomes, and improved patient satisfaction. Electronic medical records, the SBAR hand-off technique, and safety checklists are examples of standardized communication tools.

Interdisciplinary Team Collaboration

Interdisciplinary rounding can provide an opportunity for team collaboration after a patient's surgery. Much like a clear hand-off process, interdisciplinary rounds reduce patient care errors, decrease mortality rates, and improve patient outcomes. Interdisciplinary rounds are an excellent place to discuss social service needs, nutritional care services, and transportation needs with all teams coordinating care for the patient in a single setting.

The patient's service needs may vary in depth for the inpatient stay and at the time of discharge; however, there should be an evaluation of these needs and a coordination of care for those services in which there is a need. Nurses document the action plan as it relates to services and requirements for the patient and collaborate with members of the interdisciplinary team to see that next steps are executed in a timely fashion. In many instances, rounding may not be possible due to the rapid pace and turnover of the perioperative environment, and thus, clear documentation will be an absolute must to allow for synchronous care coordination.

Perioperative nurses and surgeons bring a unique skill set to the table. Perception of power between these two professionals can sometimes create a stressful environment that can also affect patient outcomes. The ability of each one to collaborate with the other is imperative so that patient safety does not become an issue. Collaboration involves joint decision-making activities between both disciplines rather than nurses only following physician orders. Although each role may have a particular focus throughout the assessment and plan of care activities, they must jointly come together to formulate the best possible treatment plan throughout the perioperative period. Studies show that an attentive communication style between nurses and physicians has the most positive impact on patients.

Ongoing education of physicians and nurses in perioperative settings may be a necessity to support a collaborative environment. In addition to continuing education and in-services, job shadowing, which exposes both the nurse and physician to each one's role, can assist in promoting understanding and teamwork.

Transfer of Care Criteria

Once a patient is ready for transfer to the **post-anesthesia care unit (PACU)**, the perioperative nurse will complete hand-off documentation and a report. Toolkits, policies, and procedures that the unit implements and utilizes should be those that a multidisciplinary team has come together to create. Various members of the interdisciplinary team must take an active role in identifying the structure and process for transferring a patient. Members of this team may include:

- Nurses (e.g., perianesthesia, perioperative, or critical care)
- Physicians (e.g., resident or surgeon)
- Allied professional team (e.g., radiology or certified surgical tech)
- Other licensed professionals (e.g., social worker or physician's assistant)
- Support staff (e.g., patient care assistant or unit clerk)
- This multidisciplinary team can help ensure that various perspectives are integrated into any standard or guideline put into place for the unit.

Communicate Current Patient Status

Interdisciplinary communication ensures patient safety. Although documentation in the EMR provides quick access to the patient's clinical history, any immediate concerns should be verbally communicated to the appropriate provider. The interdisciplinary team is composed of professionals within various disciplines and specialties. The nurse must be knowledgeable of the roles and responsibilities of each health care team member to ensure purposeful communication.

During the preoperative stage, the nurse performs a health history assessment on the patient. Information such as the patient's allergies, medications, acute and chronic illnesses, past surgeries, and overall health status must be obtained. Relevant history must be communicated to the appropriate heath care provider. The relevancy depends on the procedure.

For example, a patient with a fractured tibia will undergo internal fixation with implanted hardware. The procedure will require intraoperative imaging studies with the use of contrast media. The patient reports an allergy to shellfish during the health history assessment. The nurse must document this information in the patient's medical record and inform the surgical team prior to the procedure. The patient also reports adverse effects to general anesthesia during a past surgery. The nurse would communicate this concern to the anesthesiologist. Additionally, the patient's latest laboratory results indicate a potassium level of 6.8 mmol/L. The nurse identifies this result as a critical value. Hyperkalemia can result in cardiac arrest and must be corrected prior to surgery. Postoperatively, the nurse must continue to communicate the patient's health status with the interdisciplinary team. For example, after surgery, the patient has episodes of hypotension and verbalizes dizziness when sitting upright. A consult to physical therapy has been ordered. Before the physical therapist can assess the patient, the nurse must communicate the patient's hypotensive episodes and weight bearing status.

Communication with the interdisciplinary team must be relevant and succinct. The use of SBAR (situation-background-assessment-recommendation) can guide nurses to communicate concerns effectively. *Situation* provides a brief statement of the current problem. *Background* should include pertinent information that relates to the current situation. *Assessment* can include physical findings, lab results, objective, and subjective data. *Recommendation* is a request for resources, medications, or further guidance. For example, a patient who had abdominal surgery has end stage renal disease and is being managed by a hospitalist, nephrologist, and general surgeon. Postoperatively, the patient develops fluid volume overload. The nurse would contact the patient's nephrologist to communicate the patient's condition. Following the SBAR technique, the nurse would include the following information: "The patient recently had abdominal surgery and has developed symptoms of fluid overload. The patient has history of end stage renal disease and currently has +3 edema to the extremities and crackles upon auscultation. Should a diuretic be anticipated?"

Hand-Off Communication

The communication experience during the hand-off process should be a work of art that demonstrates all of the characteristics of a clean exchange of information among professionals. **Hand-offs** not only allow for the dissemination of information from one profession to another but serve as an opportunity for the receiving professional to ask questions and identify concerns. They act as a means to protect the patient from harm and enable professionals to provide a high level of continuity of care.

Patients are most susceptible to an adverse event during the hand-off time frame, as with most transitions in care during the perioperative period.

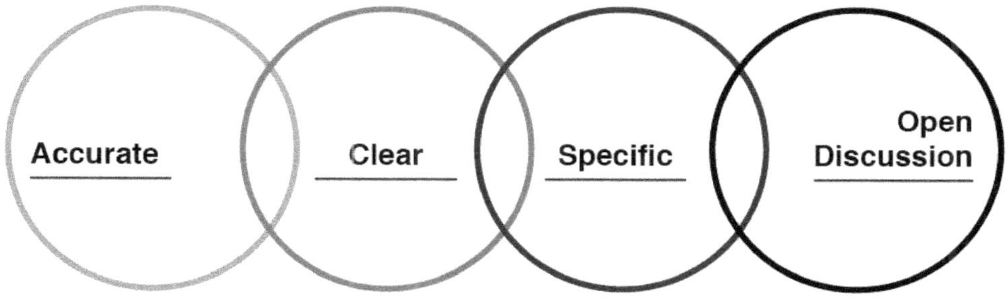

The reasons for the enhanced risk are closely related to organizational behavior and patterns during the perioperative process that may influence the hand-off process. Common distractions that arise include patient volume in the receiving unit, the need to maintain a rapid and "efficient" pace during the turnover phase, and reduction of abrasion with surgeons.

The hectic pace of the perioperative environment increases the risk for mistakes and inexplicable communication errors. According to one study, sentinel events occur as a result of poor communication practices that take place during the hand-off process. Nurses can become complacent in this exercise because it is very much part of their routine activities. Organizations must follow a standardized method for hand-off communications to reduce the danger of any impact to patient safety. This standardized approach is a requirement of The Joint Commission.

The requirement dictates that professionals must allow adequate time to exchange information and ask questions and to allow for responses. The benefit of following a standard practice helps to reduce errors and potentially avoid exclusion of pertinent data. Nurses can follow a consistent method for:

- Documentation practices
- Review and discussion of critical information
- Adequate preparation and delivery of patient care

SBAR

The **SBAR technique** is a highly favored method that nurses utilize for hand-offs. SBAR stands for Situation, Background, Assessment, and Recommendation. The advantages of using SBAR include:

- Enhancement of situational awareness
- Promotion and utilization of critical-thinking skills
- Predictable and reliable communication
- Provision of a framework that reduces bias commonly seen with organizational hierarchy and experience
- Expansion of collaborative interactions between nurses and physicians
- Advancement of collaborative discussions in nurse-to-nurse exchanges

Situation

For the situation, the perioperative nurse identifies what is happening with the patient. The overview should be concise. It is a succinct statement of the problem. Examples of situation details include:

- Demographics (patient and surgeon names, other physicians, age, admission date, surgery date)
- Problem
- Patient stability

Background

In reviewing the background, the perioperative nurse provides information about the patient's clinical background that is applicable and relevant to the patient's current situation. He or she is answering the question, "What got us to this point?" Examples of background information details include the presentation history.

Assessment

For the assessment component, perioperative nurses should describe findings and provide an analysis of possible options and considerations. Examples of assessment details include:

- Procedure-specific assessment
- Vital signs
- Temperature (route of temperature)
- Blood pressure (e.g., cuff or arterial line)
- Monitoring
- Hemodynamic pressure
- Pulse (e.g., apical or peripheral)
- Respiratory status
- Breath sounds
- Oxygen saturation
- Mechanical ventilator settings
- End-tidal Carbon Dioxide
- Monitoring
- Lab results
- Neurological function (e.g., level of consciousness)
- Intake and output (e.g., intravenous [IV] fluids)
- Location(s) of IV access
- Pain
- Pain rating
- Sedation level
- Dressings and drains
- Condition of the skin
- Drainage (type, color, amount)
- Scores
- Scores associated with the procedure itself
- Monitors and readings (including cardiac monitor)

Recommendation

Finally, the recommendation aspect of the hand-off report should serve as a discussion among professionals about what should happen next. This discussion focuses on next steps and concerns. It is an excellent opportunity to identify if there is a need to update the plan of care or notify the surgeon or physician of any findings, medication adjustments, and pending laboratory data.

Read-Back/Repeat

Some organizations incorporate an additional R, which is known as the read-back or repeat. This extra step is where staff can read back orders to ensure that there is a mutual understanding of the need.

It is a sequential process that challenges individuals only to include pertinent and relevant data. The recipient of the information validates their understanding of the information. This clarification period gives the communicator an opportunity to clarify details if necessary or to take any essential action.

The SBAR method allows perioperative nurses to spend less time writing. This effect, in turn, increases the amount of time they can focus on patient care. Studies demonstrate that use of the SBAR technique reduces the risk of adverse events, including death, and increases communication among nursing staff. It has become an industry best practice according to The Joint Commission, and as a result, organizations use electronic tools that reflect the SBAR framework to comply with The Joint Commission on Accreditation of Healthcare Organizations' National Patient Safety Goals.

Never Event

"**Never events**" refer to errors in care that should never occur during a medical procedure, due to the catastrophic effects on patient safety and outcomes that the event could have. Additionally, these events can be costly for the healthcare facility. "Never events" include instances like performing an incorrect procedure on a patient, performing a procedure on the wrong patient, failing to take into account patient history such as allergies, the development of pressure ulcers on patients in care, and other situations that cause adverse outcomes, including death, to the patient. Associated costs with "never events" include time, labor, and money spent to correct medical errors, lawsuits, and future reimbursements lost due to tarnished reputation.

Standardized Communication Plan

Standardized communication plans are a component of National Patient Safety Goals. Clear verbal, non-verbal, and written communication between healthcare providers is essential for patients to receive high quality care. Communication is especially crucial during patient transitions, such as nursing shift changes, as these periods are when patients are most likely to experience adverse outcomes. The Joint Commission recommends the SBAR communication technique when one healthcare provider is sharing information about the patient to any other provider. SBAR stands for Situation (why the communication is taking place), Background (the status and medical history of the patient), Assessment (the speaker's perspective of the problem), and Recommendation (what action the speaker believes would be most beneficial to the patient).

WHO Checklist

The World Health Organization (WHO) has published a surgical safety checklist to serve as a baseline for all medical facilities that offer surgeries. It accounts for periods that are at risk for increased or significant medical errors during perioperative period and encourages medical facilities to adapt the guidelines as needed while still addressing these critical timeframes. This document provides a standardized list of actions that should be performed in order to keep surgery patients safe.

Education of all perioperative staff, including physicians, is critical in attaining and sustaining success for SBAR to be useful.

S

Situation

I am calling about ....

The patient's Code status is ....

The problem I am calling about is ....

e.g. I am concerned the patient is going to arrest

I have just assessed the patient personally:

Vital signs are:	Blood Pressure	.... /	Pulse	....
	Respiration	....	Temperature	....

I am concerned about the:

Blood pressure because it is	**over 200** or	**less than 100** or	**30 mmHg below usual**
Pulse because it is	**over 130** or	**less than 40 and symptomatic**	
Respiration because it is	**less than 8** or	**over 30**	
Temperature because it is	**less than 96** or	**over 104**	
Urine output because it is	**less than 25 ml/hr** or	**200 ml/8hrs**	
O_2 because it is	**less than 88% on 6/liters**	**nasal cannula**	

Other ....

B

Background

The patient's mental status is:

Alert and oriented to person, place, and time

Confused and	cooperative or	non-cooperative
Agitated or	combative	

Lethargic but conversant and able to swallow

Stuporous and not talking clearly and possibly not able to swallow

Comatose	Eyes closed	Not responding to stimulation

The skin is:

Warm and dry	Pale	Mottled
Diaphoretic	Extremities are cold	Extremities are warm

The patient **is not or** **is on oxygen**

The patient has been on .... (l/min) or (5) oxygen for .... minutes (hours)

The oximeter is reading .... %

The oximeter does not detect a good pulse and is giving erratic readings.

A

Assessment

This is what I think the problem is ....

"Say what you think the problem is"

The problem seems to be cardiac infection neurologic respiratory

I am not sure what the problem is but the patient is deteriorating

The patient seems to be unstable and may get worse, we need to do something

R

Recommendation

From Physician ....

Transfer the patient to Critical Care	Come to see the patient at this time
Talk to the patient or family about Code status	Ask a consultant to see patient now

Are any tests needed:

Do you need any test like CXR ABG EKG CBC BMP

Others ....

If a change in treatment is ordered then ask:

How often do you want vital signs?

How long do you expect this problem will last?

If the patient does not get better when would you want us to call again?

Documenting Perioperative Education

Patient education during the perioperative period is imperative to achieving successful health outcomes. Documentation of the educational activities provides a record regarding the patient's understanding of the teaching and identifies gaps in knowledge. Any deficiencies should be addressed throughout the surgical experience and included in the nursing care plan as potential diagnoses. The educational concepts vary at every perioperative stage.

During the preoperative phase, the nurse performs an admission interview to evaluate the patient's knowledge of the exercises and physical activities that will be required after surgery. For example, the nurse may introduce the use of an incentive spirometer to prevent atelectasis, leg exercises to prevent blood clots, and early mobility to prevent pressure ulcers. The nurse then evaluates the patient's understanding by using a teach-back method, where the patient demonstrates the techniques they were taught.

In the intraoperative phase, the nurse orients the patient to the operating room, educating them on medications to be administered and equipment to be used. In the holding area, patients should be educated on the purposes of skin preparation and intravenous lines and fluids.

Postoperatively, the nurse re-emphasizes preoperative teaching, including early ambulation, pain management, and the need for frequent vital signs. Depending on the type of procedure, the nurse may initiate early teaching on dressing changes, catheter care, and drain management. Education is also provided to the patient's family to ensure continuity of care after discharge.

Documentation should include the concept being taught, demonstration of the activity, and the patient's understanding of the teaching. The nurse also re-evaluates the nursing care plan to ensure knowledge deficits have been addressed.

Discharge Planning and Follow Up

Discharge planning for the patient leaving the facility begins with the decision that the patient needs to have a surgical procedure. Patients who have comorbid conditions or are a part of the elderly population are at greater risk for postoperative surgical complications. Discharge planning is a fundamental component of reducing the risk of this complication and readmission. Discharge planning requires a multidisciplinary approach that may be spearheaded by the perioperative nurse. It is important to note that discharge can take place from an inpatient unit or at a facility.

Thanks to shorter hospital stays, the duration in which a nurse has to educate the patient about post-discharge care is also limited. Office-based perioperative staff, or those perioperative nurses who work in ambulatory facilities, provide education before and after surgery. Typically, education of the patient and family should take place in the days leading up to the surgery to reduce anxiety. Helping patients and families to understand what to expect the day of surgery and the days following surgery is valuable for the patient, the family, and the perioperative team.

Patient education before discharge is imperative, as studies show that timely discharge education contributes to:

- Reduction in readmissions
- Decrease in post-discharge complications

- Improvement in quality of care at the hospital and at home
- Increase in patient satisfaction
- Increase in adherence to self-care activities after discharge
- General reduction in the overall cost of care

Perioperative nurses managing patients who are undergoing procedures in which they discharge directly from a facility (as opposed to a unit) should prepare to educate patients and their families and provide for enough time to answer questions. Many organizations use a standardized set of education tools, and thus nurses should familiarize themselves with the content as well as be aware of those questions that patients and their families commonly ask.

Patients and patients' families who do not receive adequate education are at an increased risk for postoperative complications, poor symptom management, inadequate nutritional intake, substandard wound care, erratic sleep patterns, and limited activity, and they may also suffer some psychological impact.

Education that the patient and families receive may vary nonetheless as a result of the procedure, the patient, and the anesthesia. Instructions should include content that concentrates on activities of daily living, such as walking, eating, lifting, fluid intake, and wound care.

Written Postoperative Discharge Instructions for Lumbar Spine Surgery	
Nutrition	• Return to your diet slowly. • Initially, you may want to avoid foods that are spicy.
Activity	• Avoid strenuous activity for the next six weeks. • Avoid lifting objects greater than ten pounds for the next six weeks or twisting or bending. • Take short walks for the next four to six weeks that last ten to fifteen minutes in duration, and then slowly increase time until, by week six, you are walking upwards of one hour. • Avoid use of exercise equipment such as treadmills, stair climbers, or elliptical trainers unless cleared by your physician. • Discuss increasing your activity schedule with your physician. • You are permitted to shower the following day; however, cover the surgical site with plastic so that it stays dry. • Baths, pools, or Jacuzzis are not allowed. • Avoid sitting for greater than thirty minutes for meals. • Try to sit in a reclining position. • When lying down, a pillow between the legs may greatly increase your level of comfort. • Sexual activities may resume within the next seven days; however, your role should be passive. A side-lying or back position is best.
Getting out of Bed	• Ensure that you are lying flat, and then roll sideways, and push your body up.

Written Postoperative Discharge Instructions for Lumbar Spine Surgery	
Wound Care	• Do not remove your dressing until tomorrow. • If your dressing gets wet, remove it, and cover it with a dry dressing. • Change dressing daily. • Apply ice to the lower back region for ten to twenty minutes each day for four days. DO NOT PLACE ICE DIRECTLY ON SKIN. Cover the ice pack with a pillow slip. • Call the doctor if you see any drainage on the dressing.
Medications	• Be sure to take pain medications as prescribed for the first thirty-six to seventy-two hours to reduce risk of pain symptoms. • Stool softeners may be taken to prevent constipation. • Resume taking medications as prescribed by your physician. • Avoid taking any medications that contain aspirin for a minimum of four days.
When to Call the Doctor	Call the doctor if: • You have excessive drainage around the surgical site • You experience a temperature greater than 101 degrees (Fahrenheit) • You have any tenderness or swelling around the surgical site • You have unexplained shortness of breath, anxiety, or sweating • You have pain that is not relieved by medication

Collaboration

Continued collaboration between patients and a representative of their healthcare team promotes positive recovery outcomes. Patients who are contacted regularly after discharge to review their health, medical records, instructions, and satisfaction are less likely to experience poor recovery or be readmitted to the medical facility. Additionally, nurses who collaborate with other health professionals to create patient discharge plans are also associated with improved patient outcomes. This correlation is likely due to input from a variety of medical perspectives that allows the discharge plan to address all potential patient needs.

Health Literacy

Health literacy refers to how capable patients are of understanding their diagnosis, treatment plans, prognosis, and follow-up health instructions. A high degree of health literacy is associated with the ability to make personal health decisions, higher confidence in personal health decisions, and higher compliance with medical instructions.

Pain Management

Pain management is a vital component of discharge care. Not only does the patient need to be comfortable, but it is also important that they receive correct medication, dosing, and follow safe guidelines for any therapeutic recommendations. Patients may not be able to effectively manage their pain if they fail to follow dosing instructions of prescription medications. They may inadvertently engage in unsafe behavior if they do not follow limitations of certain prescription medications. For example, opioids are highly addictive and make routine behaviors, such as driving a vehicle, dangerous. Therefore, it is crucial that pain management counseling is provided as a part of discharge services. Following up with patients who have documented pain and management techniques may also mitigate risks. This practice can additionally allow nurses to review and modify pain management plans as patient needs change over time, while also noticing if there are any early causes for concern.

Postoperative Follow-Up

Perioperative staff will conduct telephonic follow-up calls to assess for any postoperative problems, including any changes in health status, medication regimen validation, and verification of appointment; address patient or caregiver concerns; and provide additional education. Also, additional coordination of services such as home services may require support at this time. Patients and families receive reinforcement education about what to do should any health or medical issues arise during the recovery period.

The postoperative follow-up call can also be a time in which the nurse can determine if there is any risk or signs of nonadherence behaviors, as these may sometimes emerge during the conversation. Such patients may require follow-up by home health services for further education or other support services, such as transportation to appointments or pharmacy mail order program information.

The perioperative staff conducting the call should verify contact information before the patient's discharge and if there is a need for translation services. Meanwhile, if the nurse identifies any discrepancies with the patient's recovery, an additional call may be necessary.

Nurses must document postoperative follow-up calls in the patient's medical record. Documentation allows for tracking of patient progress but also enables the treating health care institution to monitor for outcomes. Nurses should also document communication with physicians about any adverse findings during the postoperative call.

Transfer of Care Documentation and Reporting

When possible, a face-to-face discussion will take place between the team transferring the patient and the staff receiving the patient. A patient qualifies for transfer to a different unit once their health status stabilizes and transfer of care does not create a safety risk. Perioperative nurses must document all transfers of care within the patient's medical record.

Here is an example of an SBAR intraoperative hand-off to the PACU:

Components of an Intraoperative SBAR Hand-Off to PACU	
Situation	• Patient name • Surgical Procedure (including site) • Anesthetist provider name • Surgeon name
Background	• Anesthesia administration • Medications and dosage (including antibiotics) • IV fluids/sites • Blood type/products • Specimens (type, location, quantity, tests requested) • Estimated blood loss • Urine output • Surgical sites • Dressings, tubes, drainage (including location) • Unexpected or adverse events in the OR
Assessment	• Hemodynamic stability • Respiratory/airway/oxygenation status • Pain status and pain management • Body temperature (i.e., hyperthermia or hypothermia) • Neuro status • Monitoring (equipment, lines) • Special needs (e.g., autism, disabilities) • Safety risks
Recommendations	• Implement postoperative orders • Allow for time to answer questions of PACU staff before, during, and after transfer of patient • Actively support patient transfer activities (including lines, equipment, and patient) • Address any known family concerns • Discharge from the PACU once stable

Regulatory Requirements for Tracking Equipment Provided by External Sources

In the OR, there may be an occasional need for equipment, instruments, or other items to be brought in, or loaned from an outside source. As an example, a hospital system may comprise several different hospitals in one city, and products or other essential surgical items may be shared among facilities should the need arise. Generally, transfers or loans involving instrumentation or supplies will be coordinated by the OR manager or specialty leader, central sterile supply departments, and chosen couriers. Log sheets should be used to track the item, time and date of arrival/departure, name of the staff member logging the item, and where the item originated. If the item is an instrument or non-disposable item, sterilization will be required upon arrival to the borrowing facility, and a designated tag or label should remain with the instrument so as to differentiate it as a loaner.

Equipment loaned from an outside source will usually arrive through the logistics department and will require a maintenance check by biomedical personnel prior to use. It is important that the perioperative staff members receiving the equipment check for the preventative maintenance tag (placed by the biomedical personnel) and for a loaner tag of some sort. Borrowed equipment should also be documented on a log sheet for easier tracking.

Supplies or implanted devices may also be brought in from the outside via a vendor or from another hospital's supply. Usually this should be coordinated in advance of the surgery, but occasionally there will be an urgent need due to time and low supply of essential items. It is imperative that these items are not new to the hospital system and that the products have been approved through the facility's analysis committee. This approval process is a multidisciplinary effort among logistics management, materials management, OR management, and upper hospital management and may differ among hospital systems.

Any special instructions regarding package handling or sterilization parameters must be included with the items or communicated to the perioperative nurse or central sterile supply manager. As with any supply or device in the OR, the perioperative staff must inspect the integrity of packaging and be cognizant of expiration dates.

Facilitating Transfer to the Next Level of Care

After completion of the procedure, the provider and/or surgeon will give orders for the patient to be transferred to the next level of care. The determination of where the patient is transferred is dependent on several factors, including intraoperative complications, patient acuity, and hemodynamic stability. Perioperative nurses must anticipate a post-surgical transfer to the intensive care unit (ICU) or post anesthesia care unit (PACU).

Any patient who has received anesthesia during surgery must be monitored postoperatively in a unit equipped to perform frequent assessments and emergency interventions. Priority assessments in the PACU include oxygenation, level of consciousness, and cardiovascular status. The patient's respiratory status must be assessed continuously to ensure an intact airway. Assessments include respiratory rate, depth, rhythm, breath sounds, and oxygen saturation levels. Level of consciousness includes the patient's alertness and ability to follow commands. Cardiovascular status is assessed via vital signs, cardiac monitoring, and temperature. The nurse observes trends, compares them to the patient's baseline, and reports any deviations from the norm. Patient criteria for transfer out of the PACU is often included in hospital protocols. Once the patient meets the criteria, they can be transferred safely to an inpatient unit or be discharged home. Most patients transferred to the PACU remain on the unit for approximately one hour postoperatively.

In some instances, the patient will become unstable during the procedure and require a transfer to the ICU. Other patients have extensive surgeries or medical conditions requiring constant monitoring. Patients who are unstable or need to remain intubated benefit from ICU care. The nurse must anticipate critical care orders by the provider. For example, if a patient was unable to spontaneously breathe on their own after general anesthesia, the patient will remain intubated. The patient will require mechanical ventilation in the immediate postoperative period. The patient would be transferred to ICU for continued care.

Regulatory Guidelines

HIPAA

The **Health Insurance Portability and Accountability Act of 1996** (**HIPAA**) aims to keep patient health records confidential and secure, allows individuals to conditionally keep employer-sponsored health insurance for a certain period of time should they leave a job, and standardizes electronic processes relating to healthcare services. All healthcare providers and health insurance providers in the United States must follow the guidelines established in HIPAA.

Regulatory Agency

A regulatory agency is an entity established and operated by the federal, state, or local government in which it resides. Regulatory agencies establish standard operating procedures, rules, and benchmarks by which business organization in a particular industry must comply. Almost all industries that provide goods or services to public populations are governed in some way by a regulatory agency. Common regulatory agencies that medical facilities work with include the Centers for Disease Control and Prevention (CDC) (which focuses on public health initiatives and best practices), the **Food and Drug Administration** (**FDA**) (which focuses on safe manufacturing practices relating to food and pharmaceutical production and transport), the Agency for Health Research and Quality (which researches and establishes guidelines relating to quality), and the Centers for Medicare and Medicaid Services (which oversee all administrative processes for facilities that accept reimbursements from the Medicare and Medicaid programs).

Read-Back for Verbal Orders

Read-back occurs when staff reads back orders to ensure that there is a mutual understanding of the need. It is a sequential process that challenges individuals to include only pertinent and relevant data. The recipient of the information validates their understanding of the information. This clarification period gives the communicator an opportunity to clarify details if necessary or to take any essential action.

Ideally, verbal orders should only occur when the provider is physically unable to write out the orders due to an emergency or other extenuating circumstances. Verbal orders must be carefully read back to the provider to ensure accuracy. The verbal order process includes receiving, reading back, documenting, and executing the order. During the read-back, the nurse must repeat the order that was given as it is interpreted. The provider must then confirm the read-back with the nurse.

After the verbal order has been given, the nurse must document the date and time of the order as well as the provider's name. After the emergency situation has passed, the provider must review the verbal order for accuracy and sign the order, including the date and time. Verbal orders must be physically signed by the provider within 24 hours of being given to the nurse.

Surgical Wound Classifications

Documentation of the surgical wound class occurs immediately after the procedure. If the surgical wound class is not properly identified, an SSI may be improperly labeled as "hospital-acquired." Centers for Medicare and Medicaid Services (CMS) may withhold reimbursement to healthcare facilities and providers based on hospital acquired conditions such as SSI.

Surgical wound classification is based on the degree of contamination. Classification of wounds determines the type of treatment that is required to maintain the wound free of infection and promote recovery. There are four classifications of wounds.

Class I wounds are considered clean. A clean wound is a surgical incision that has not penetrated cavities, such as the lungs or urinary tract, and has been performed under sterile conditions. Class I wounds carry the least risk of infection. An example of a class I wound is excision of a lipoma.

Class II wounds are classified as clean-contaminated. Class II wounds are those that involve organs or internal tissues under sterile conditions. Any opening in the skin carries a risk of infection. Although surgeries are performed in a sterile environment, the risk of contamination for class II wounds is higher. An example of a class II wound is an open cholecystectomy.

Class III wounds are considered contaminated. Contaminated wounds result from non-sterile technique, such as a thoracotomy in the emergency department. The risk of infection is high, and the nurse should anticipate continuous monitoring for signs and symptoms of infection.

Class IV wounds carry the highest risk of infection. These wounds are considered dirty-infected. Class IV wounds are usually infected prior to the surgical procedure, such as a gangrenous diabetic ulcer. Alternatively, surgical wounds that repair perforated organs are also considered class IV wounds. For example, an exploratory laparotomy due to bowel perforation causing peritonitis is considered a class IV wound.

Practice Quiz

1. Which of the following is the correct description of SBAR?
    a. Situation, background, assessment, recommendation
    b. Status, background, adjustment, risk
    c. Scores, background, assessment, risk factors
    d. Standards, background, adequacy, recommendation

2. Which of the following is NOT a benefit of using SBAR?
    a. Perioperative nurses spend an excessive amount of time writing, but they are able to draw attention to adverse events using this process.
    b. Perioperative nurses are able to focus on patient care.
    c. The SBAR process increases communication among members of the perioperative staff.
    d. SBAR eliminates the need for face-to-face communication.

3. Which of the following is the correct description of I PASS?
    a. I PASS is an interview technique that perioperative nurses use in the outpatient setting.
    b. I PASS is an acronym that stands for introduction, patient, assessment, situation, and safety concerns.
    c. I PASS is an example of an IT system that promotes efficiency in the perioperative environment.
    d. I PASS is a checklist that the World Health Organization implemented in 2007 to improve the efficiency of discharge planning.

4. When is the best time to raise a concern about a procedure that a patient has undergone?
    a. Before the surgery or procedure begins
    b. During the surgery or procedure
    c. Immediately following the surgery or procedure
    d. Before, during, and after a surgery or procedure

5. Which of the following can be a barrier to communication?
    a. Quiet environment
    b. New computer technology and applications
    c. Low turnover productivity standards
    d. Prioritizing during documentation

See answers on next page.

Answer Explanations

1. A: SBAR is an acronym that stands for situation, background, assessment, and recommendation. It is a process that allows for a structured hand-off between nurses, allowing for the ability to have a collaborative discussion while also creating awareness of the patient's current health status and potential risks.

2. D: The SBAR technique is a best practice that allows nurses to focus on providing patient care because it decreases the amount of time they spend writing. Also, the design of this process promotes open communication among the perioperative nursing team. SBAR can be used face-to-face or by telephone, and it should always be a verbal conversation.

3. B: I PASS is a technique that is similar to the SBAR technique. Perioperative teams may use this technique to promote a standardized method for information exchange during the hand-off process.

4. D: Perioperative nursing staff should escalate concerns to the surgeon, treating physician, and other perioperative staff any time there is a risk for an adverse or poor outcome to the patient.

5. B: New technology and limited understanding of the new technology can prove to be a barrier to communication for staff who are unable to access information, document patient data, or share results with fellow perioperative staff. The surroundings may also prove to be a detriment to effective communication (i.e., alarms, high volume, and rapid turnover). Nurses should prioritize the appropriate time to document and which information to document; this allows for smoother workflow and allocates time for communication.

Infection Prevention and Control

Environmental Cleaning

The practice of environmental cleaning considers all influences in a medical setting that could reduce or eliminate the spread of infection or disease to patients. Medical settings are exposed to a variety of pathogens on a regular basis, and the majority of patients in these settings are immunocompromised to some degree. Therefore, stringent cleaning protocols of areas that are frequented by medical staff, auxiliary staff, and patients must be established and diligently followed. Most hospitals and other medical settings use chemical disinfectants, visual inspections, standardized behavioral protocol (such as hand sanitizing upon entering or leaving patient rooms), and other quality processes to maintain environmental cleanliness.

Environmental Management

Given the importance of sterile integrity in the OR, the circulator (circulating nurse) must ensure that the overall environment is safe for staff and patients. One potential issue is a spill of hazardous liquids in the OR, especially blood. The circulator should always follow universal protocols when dealing with bodily fluids, and in the event of a spill, the circulator should cautiously ensure the spill is addressed promptly by the appropriate personnel.

One of the most common management challenges is room turnover. In order to keep the OR schedule running smoothly, the turnover times must be effectively managed. If turnover times are extended unnecessarily, it may start a chain reaction of delayed cases, which impacts the operational and financial performance. However, there also should be a balance between expediting case turnover and OR protocols. For example, the trash and used equipment, instruments, and materials should stay in the room until the procedure is completed in the event of an incorrect count.

Each facility may have its own protocol for terminal cleaning, and the circulator should be aware of the schedule for terminal cleaning and assist as necessary. One of the main goals of terminal cleaning is to eliminate all dust in the OR, including the dust and debris that may be missed with regular cleaning. Stationary equipment should be moved to ensure that contaminants that may be underneath the equipment are cleaned and disinfected. Tasks for terminal cleaning may include moving all equipment from the room to clean walls and floors and thorough cleaning of the OR table, positioning equipment, overhead lights, anesthesia equipment, and computer equipment.

Cleaning and Disinfecting Instruments

Perioperative scrub personnel are responsible for cleaning instruments during and immediately following an operative procedure. There is an expectation that this team will follow disinfectant and sterilization procedures to protect the safety of patients and fellow health care workers. Failure to follow proper procedures can lead to disastrous outcomes.

Health care facilities follow the Occupational Safety and Health Administration (OSHA) regulations and the Association of perioperative Registered Nurses (AORN) practice guidelines for cleaning instruments.

Contaminating organisms, known as bioburdens or biofilms, can accumulate on the surfaces and within the crevices, ports, or other components of a device during a procedure. They are not easy to remove and require oxidizing chemicals to do so. To prevent debris from sticking to surfaces, instruments, or within channels, sterile water flushes or irrigation can help to keep channels and instrument surfaces clean.

Instruments must undergo the process of bioburden or contaminating organisms' removal before sterilization or disinfection. Saline should never be utilized to support this process because it can cause mineral deposits to form within or on the instrument. The use of saline can create pitting or even lead to corrosion. Once clean, the device is ready to undergo decontamination. An enzymatic or detergent solution is utilized to loosen the material on the instrument.

Also, there are those devices that have an automatic cleaning function for the ports of apparatuses to be flushed, allowing for a cost-effective method to clean instruments that have a reusable channel. Perioperative staff must familiarize themselves with the practice and process those instruments with this function. The U.S. FDA requires manufacturers to comply with federal, professional, and regional standards when reprocessing reusable instruments. This expectation includes the provision of written instructions for reprocessing for all reusable devices.

Some instruments will undergo decontamination using a cavitation or ultrasonic cleaning process, which entails the use of high-frequency energy that creates microscopic bubbles that remove microscopic debris.

The solution chosen to clean the instrument may vary but can prove to be extremely useful in working with the power of a cleansing device. The pH of a cleaning solution varies but has a direct impact on the cleaning power of the solution. The pH can drive the acidity, neutrality, and alkalinity of a product. If a detergent is too acidic, it can damage stainless steel instruments, leading to pitting or corrosion. Ultimately, the type of instrument requiring cleaning may determine the type of solution selected (i.e., surfactant, chelate, buffer).

AAMI

The Association for the Advancement of Medical Instrumentation (AAMI) focuses on safe medical device development, manufacturing, circulation, and reuse. This is an independent organization whose membership is voluntary; however, many healthcare and medical device manufacturing facilities embrace its quality standards as highly reputable. AAMI shares resources for organizations to develop comprehensive quality management systems. The association also establishes standards for cleanliness of and sterilization techniques for a wide range of medical instruments. These guidelines vary based on whether they are for a healthcare facility that is using and storing instruments, or a manufacturing company that builds, packages, stores, and ships them.

Sterilization and Disinfection Terminology

Sterilization is the destruction and removal of microbial life, including spores. Once something is sterile, the probability of microorganism survival is one in one million.

Disinfection involves the use of chemical agents that eliminate or kill all pathogenic microorganisms, with the exception of a high number of bacterial spores on inanimate objects. Disinfecting entails using antiseptics and germicides to destroy microorganisms.

The type of disinfectant chosen depends on the action or function that is necessary for the chemical to perform. Also, criteria such as safety, effect on equipment, cost, and impact to the environment should be taken into consideration prior to use.

Disinfectants may be split into three categories: high level, intermediate level. and low level. These categories refer to the disinfectant's capabilities.

Level of Disinfectant	Description	Solution
High-Level	High-level disinfectants kill a broad spectrum of microorganisms. However, bacterial spores can survive.	High-level disinfectants receive Food and Drug Administration (FDA) clearance. Example solutions include peracetic acid (PAA), hydrogen peroxides, glutaraldehyde, formaldehyde, and ortho-phthalaldehyde.
Intermediate-Level	Intermediate-level disinfectants kill tubercle bacilli, vegetative bacteria, many viruses, and fungi; however, bacterial spores can survive.	Intermediate-level disinfectants consist of chemical germicides that are registered as tuberculocides by the Environmental Protection Agency (EPA). Solutions consist of alcohols, hypochlorites, iodine, and iodophor disinfectants.
Low-Level	Low-level disinfectants kill vegetative bacteria, some viruses, and fungi.	Chemical germicides are registered as hospital disinfectants by the EPA. Solutions consist of phenolics or quaternary ammonium compounds.

Disinfectants can be irritating to the skin and mucous membranes. Therefore, any use of these chemicals should always take place in an environment with adequate ventilation. Vapor control systems are especially beneficial in protecting staff from irritation.

The Spaulding Classification System

The Spaulding Classification System (named for founder Earle Spaulding) classifies items that require disinfection as being critical, semicritical, or noncritical. These classifications relate to the risk of infection for the patient. Also, the level of disinfection chosen has a direct relationship with the instrument and method of utilization.

Critical Items

Critical items are those devices that enter the sterile tissue or vascular system such as catheters, implants, and ultrasound probes. They have a high risk for infection through microorganism contamination. Institutions purchase these instruments or use steam sterilization. Those instruments that are heat-sensitive receive ethylene oxide or hydrogen peroxide gas plasma.

Semicritical Items

Semicritical items are those instruments or equipment that comes in contact with mucous membranes or nonintact skin. Examples of semicritical items include laryngoscope blades, cystoscopes, and anesthesia. Although the lungs and gastrointestinal tract may not be susceptible to bacterial spore infections, they are at risk for infections resulting from bacteria, mycobacteria, and viruses. These items undergo intermediate-level disinfection using chemical disinfectants. Commonly used disinfectants for semicritical items include glutaraldehyde, hydrogen peroxide, ortho-phthalaldehyde, and PAA with hydrogen peroxide.

Endoscopes require flushing with sterile water to prevent any adverse effects that might occur with use of a disinfectant. While tap water or filtered water may also aid in flushing endoscopes and channels, there is a risk for organism contamination, and therefore, sterile water is the preference.

Forced-air drying can assist in the reduction of bacterial contamination, and therefore these items should undergo forced-air drying before they are packed and stored away.

Noncritical Items

Noncritical items are those devices that do not come in contact with mucous membranes but do come in contact with intact skin. Examples of noncritical items include bedpans, blood pressure cuffs, crutches, bedside tables, bed rails, and floors. Low-level disinfectants are appropriate for these items. Decontamination often takes place in the same location of usage. A single-use disposable towel to clean a bedside table surface is an example of surface cleaning in the physical place of use. Transmission of infectious agents to patients from noncritical items is very rare.

Categories of Sterilants and Disinfectants

Sterilants, or chemical germicides and **disinfectants**, may fall into a variety of categories. The most common two types include oxidizing agents and alkylating agents.

Oxidizing Agents

Hydrogen peroxide is not only effective in cleaning wounds, but it is also useful as a disinfectant and sterilizing agent for surgical instruments.

Accelerated hydrogen peroxide is effective in fighting against bacteria, viruses, fungi, and spores. Health institutions use it as a disinfectant. Damage to soft metals such as brass, copper, and aluminum is a risk in using accelerated hydrogen peroxide.

Peracetic acid (PAA) is a high-level disinfectant used in aseptic packaging and disinfection. It is a moderately stronger oxidizing agent than hydrogen peroxide. It is effective against bacteria, spores, yeasts, fungi, mycobacteria, and viruses and can reduce microbial populations in wounds that have contamination. PAA is a rapid-acting oxidizer that remains active at low temperatures.

Sodium hypochlorite is one of the most successful disinfecting agents in health care facilities. Low concentrations of this solution can prove to be highly useful as a powerful oxidizing disinfectant as a result of its ability to kill organisms, even with low temperatures. This characteristic makes it especially attractive to health care institutions because it can reduce the transmission of diseases.

Alkylating Agents

One method of sterilization is **gas sterilization**. Instruments undergo exposure to high concentrations of reactive gasses and vapors for a prescribed period within a sealed chamber.

Ethylene oxide sterilization is a low-temperature process in which ethylene oxide gas decreases the number of infectious agents. It is especially beneficial for those instruments that cannot endure the heat of an autoclave sterilization environment. The duration in which the process takes place may vary depending on the type of device that is undergoing sterilization; however, cycles may last between thirty-six and forty-eight hours.

Formaldehyde sterilization is most effective in a highly concentrated gaseous state. It is most useful for those instruments and medical equipment that cannot endure high-temperature sterilization. The staff that uses this method of sterilization may be subject to monitoring if they exceed exposure level limits, as this can lead to injury.

Steam Sterilization

Steam sterilization is the oldest decontamination and sterilization method that uses pressurized steam to kill microorganisms. This method of sterilization works best with those items that can withstand heat and moisture.

Steam sterilization requires temperature, time, pressure, and saturated steam to function properly. These things take place in an autoclave or a high-speed prevacuum sterilizer. Autoclaves receive steam at the top or sides of the sterilizing chamber and force the air out of the bottom of the chamber through a drain vent. High-speed prevacuum sterilizers have a vacuum pump that ensures air removal from the sterilizing chamber and loads ahead of steam admission. The prevacuum pump allows for quick steam penetration. The functionality of these machines undergoes the Bowie-Dick test each day to assess for air leaks or poor air removal and includes the use of 100 percent cotton surgical towels that are clean and preconditioned.

Another steam sterilization method is known as the steam flush-pressure pulsing process. This process involves the rapid movement of air through a repeatedly alternating flush of steam and pressure pulse above the atmosphere pressure. Sterilization duration using this method is three to four minutes at 132 to 135 degrees Celsius. The system also participates in a monitoring process much like the others in which temperature, time, and pressure measurements are reviewed.

The duration in which instruments remain in the system varies by the items requiring sterilization, type of sterilizing system in use, cycle design, bioburden, altitude, package, side, and design. End users must follow the instructions as written by the manufacturer of the sterilizer to achieve the best possible outcome.

While steam sterilization is a commonly utilized method of sterilization, there is some risk that this approach may not be as effective as necessary if it is unable to remove the biofilm adequately. There are some implants and instrument sets that require extended cycles to achieve sterilization.

Flash Sterilization

Flash sterilization is another form of sterilization that can prove useful in sterilizing critical medical devices. It is another form of steam sterilization. The item is placed on a tray and undergoes flashing with rapid steaming. This process is done in close proximity to the OR to expedite delivery to the point of service. Flash sterilization is often utilized when there is not enough time to sterilize an item by usual prepackaged methods. It should not be used for "convenience" or instances where there is a risk for infections, nor should it be used with implantable devices.

This method is associated with some adverse episodes such as infections. Also, burns from the instruments have occurred. As a result of these events, policies have been instituted to help avoid preventable burns. Patient burns are avoidable if cooling protocol are followed. Air cooling or immersion in sterile liquid can help with the cooling process.

Heat-Based Sterilization

Heat-based sterilization methods such as a steam autoclave or dry heat oven is a viable option for heat-stable, reusable medical instruments that enter the bloodstream or sterile tissue. Arthroscopic and laparoscopic telescopes should undergo sterilization before use; however, in those instances where this practice is not possible, high-level disinfection is the method of choice. Meanwhile, those components of the endoscopic set such as the trocars and operative instruments can undergo heat-based sterilization methods such as the steam autoclave or dry heat oven.

Type of Sterilization	Description
Steam Sterilization	Steam sterilization is the oldest decontamination and sterilization method that uses pressurized steam to kill microorganisms. **Advantages:** • It is a cost-effective form of sterilization. • It works best with devices that are heat and moisture tolerant.
Ethylene Oxide "Gas" Sterilization	This process is used to sterilize those instruments that are not able to withstand high steam sterilization (e.g., plastic packaging, plastic containers, and electronic components). **Advantages:** • Ability to sterilize instruments that are heat sensitive **Disadvantages:** • Cycle time • Cost • Hazards to the patient and staff
Liquid Chemical Sterilization	Liquid chemical sterilization entails the use of a chemical agent to sterilize an instrument. **Advantages:** • Rapid sterilization • Effective for heat-sensitive devices **Disadvantages:** • Cannot fully penetrate barriers such as blood, tissue, and biofilm • Viscosity of some liquids prevents them from reaching pathogens in narrow lumens • Devices may need rinsing after the liquid chemical sterilant, but the water may not be sterile

Type of Sterilization	Description
Ozone Sterilizer	Ozone oxidizes organic matter including bacteria, fungi, and viruses found on instruments. It is able to sterilize equipment at a low temperature and is easy to use. The manufacturer's instructions must be followed closely for proper use. **Advantages:** • Cost-effective • Compatible with aluminum, titanium, ceramic, glass, Teflon, and silicone containers **Disadvantages:** • May be inadequate for killing MERSA
Plasma Sterilization System	The low-temperature hydrogen peroxide gas plasma sterilization can be used with those items that are moisture and heat sensitive. It removes microbial organisms through use of hydrogen peroxide vapor and free radicals that disrupt the microbial cell membranes and enzymes. This system sterilizes instruments within thirty minutes to a little more than an hour using hydrogen peroxide gas. Users must follow the manufacturer's instructions because the system can only be used with certain instruments.
Infrared Radiation	This sterilizer destroys spores. **Advantages:** • Short cycle duration • Alternative for heat-resistant instruments **Not FDA cleared
Gaseous Chlorine Dioxide	The gaseous chlorine dioxide system is a health care sterilization system that has the capacity to sterilize instruments in a short period of time. **Not FDA cleared

Transporting and Storing Sterile Supplies

Perioperative personnel should ensure that instruments remain ready for transport at all times during and after the procedure. During the procedure, soiled instruments must continue to be moist so that a biofilm does not form during the process.

- Sterile Water Towel Wrap: Instruments remain wet by wrapping them with a damp towel that is wet with sterile water.
- Humid Package: Perioperative staff place the devices inside of a package that can sustain a moisture-rich environment. Also, an instrument spray or gel can assist in keeping biofilms from adhering to the devices.

- Presoaking: Instruments may also undergo presoaking in an enzymatic solution immediately following use. To ensure proper dilution, temperature, and soak time, perioperative personnel should follow the manufacturer's instructions.

When the time arrives for transport, perioperative staff discards these solutions. If, for any reason, the staff is not able to discard the solution used to soak the instruments, the team can pour the solution into a leak-proof container and label it as a biohazardous material. Scrub personnel must separate sharp instruments (e.g., forceps with teeth, scissors, perforating towel clamps, and curettes) from more delicate instruments to avoid punctures or damage. The team must place contaminated, disposable sharp instruments into a puncture-resistant container that is leak-proof, closed, and labeled as a biohazard. Also, lighter or more delicate instruments should lie on top of the heavier tools to prevent damage.

Transportation of Containers and Carts

Staff must transport contaminated instruments in bins with lids or within enclosed carts that are large enough to hold the devices. These transport containers must be leak-proof and puncture-resistant and have a biohazard label or be easily distinguishable as a biohazardous container. Sharp instruments or those items with sharp borders and edges are transported in puncture-proof containers to prevent injury to others.

Some facilities may use carts and containers that carry clean instruments to the location of the procedure and then use the same cart to transport contaminated instruments after the procedure. These carts must also wear biohazard labels once there is any placement of contaminated instruments in the vehicle.

Documentation

Documentation Required for Monitoring Safe Sterilization Practices

The sterilization process requires the documentation of key chemical indicators (CIs), process challenge devices (PCDs), and biological indicators (BIs) that indicate testing has taken the place of sterilizers, and these sterilization records should be kept on file as a demonstration of compliance with Joint Commission standards for a period of three years.

Those who participate in the sterilization process must be knowledgeable about what critical information to record and how to record it. This information should be available within departmental procedures or from the manufacturer.

Documentation of sterility practices allows for tracking of sterilizer performance. Four elements that define the effectiveness of a sterility assurance program include:

- Consistent load release for implant and nonimplant loads
- Sterilizer qualification testing
- Consistent sterilizer efficacy monitoring
- Product quality assurance testing

Documentation Practices for Continuous Quality Improvement

Documentation not only ensures consistency and accuracy in sterilization practices, but it can also serve to facilitate opportunities for process improvements. For example, daily sterilization testing practices might change to testing before each load if documentation shows sterilization failures occurring at a high rate. Trending data can prove useful in supporting decisions to change a process or possibly even shift the maintenance practices.

Safe Handling Practices

Hazardous/Biohazardous Materials

Safe handling of hazardous and biohazardous materials is a critical function of perioperative staff. Universal-, standard-, and transmission-based precautions each enable perioperative staff to adhere to a set of standards that were designed to prevent and protect staff from the transmission of blood-borne infections or diseases.

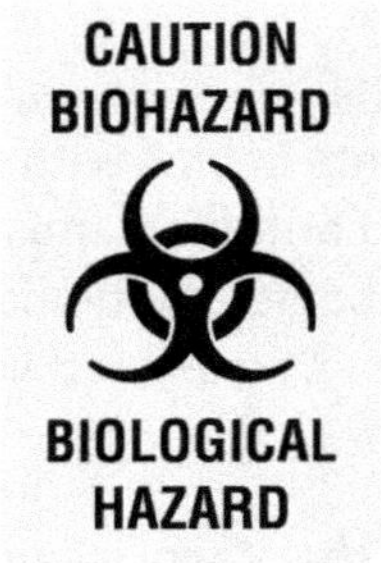

OSHA requires organizations to develop exposure protocol plans that are shared with perioperative staff and undergo a review and revision on an annual basis.

Best practices must be implemented and followed to reduce the risk of employee exposure, which may include a core set of processes and procedures that address:

- Specimen storage and transportation to include warning labels
- Use of personal protective equipment (PPE) and employer provision of those items including gloves, gowns, and masks
- Management of contaminated needles (i.e., not recapping used needles)
- Signage in plain view with biohazard logos
- Housekeeping schedule creation and posting
- Management of contaminated laundry

Use standard precautions for the care of all patients

Standard precautions apply to:
- blood non-intact skin ▪ mucous membranes
- all body fluids, secretions and excretions except sweat

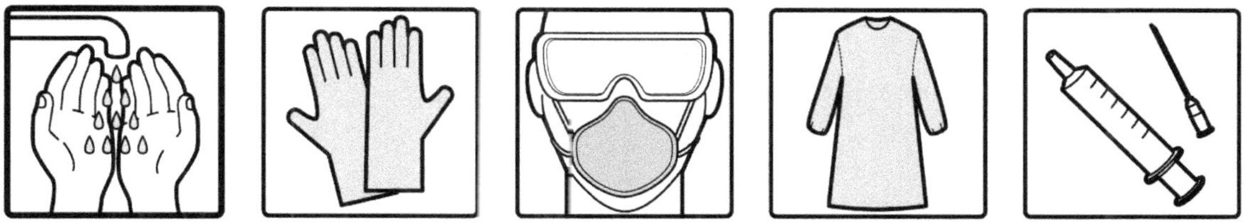

Wash hands	Wear gloves	Wear mask	Wear gown	Sharp disposal
Wash hands properly and thoroughly between patient contact and other contact with body fluids or soiled equipment.	Wear gloves when handling blood, body fluids, nonintact skin or soiled items. Change gloves between patients. Wash hands after removing gloves.	Wear a mask and eye protection or face shield to protect mucous membranes of the eyes, nose, and mouth when likely to be splashed.	Wear a gown to protect skin and prevent soiling of clothing when likely to be splashed or spayed. Wash hands after removing gown	Dispose of syringes and other sharps into a designated closed container. **Do not** break or bend needles.

Follow established policies and procedures for patient placement, environmental controls, patient-care equipment, and linen

Safe Handling of Chemotherapeutic Agents

Perioperative nursing staff may care for patients with cancer at some point in their treatment. They are not generally required to administer IV chemotherapy because this is a function typically managed by a physician or oncology nurse. The surgeon may administer chemotherapy in the OR during the surgical procedure, or this may take place following the procedure in another location. However, perioperative nurses may have to handle these chemotherapeutic agents.

Chemotherapeutic Agent	Medication Class	Route of Administration in the Perioperative Setting
Biodegradable Polymers	Alkylating agent	Intracranial, intracavity
Methotrexate	Antimetabolite	Intrathecal
Mitomycin	Antineoplastic antibiotic	Intravesical instillation, topical ophthalmic
Cytarabine	Antimetabolite	Intrathecal
Pegaspargase	Enzyme	Intramuscular injection

These agents can be a hazard to perioperative nurses who are handling them due to the antineoplastic agents, which are toxic compounds. Therefore, these agents require special handling and disposal. They have the label of being on the "P-list" or "U-list." These lists help to identify which commercial chemical products are "hazardous." There are three items or sets of criteria that must be met for an agent to receive the designation of P or U.

Criteria for P or U Designation

- The formulation has to contain a chemical on the P- or U-list.
- The chemical in the waste must be unused.
- The chemical in the waste has to be the only active ingredient.

Evidence-based practices for safe handling of chemotherapeutic agents are imperative for the safety of staff. Processes and procedures should address items such as:

- Appropriate use of PPE
- Transportation and disposal procedures
- Sterile processing
- Documentation protocol for chemotherapy
- Acceptable environment preparation of chemotherapeutic agents
- Physician orders
- Medication safety and chemotherapy time-out

Process	Description
Appropriate Use of PPE	Perioperative personnel and physicians should don appropriate PPE during chemotherapy procedures that take place within the perioperative setting. Proper practices should include: • Double gloving • Wearing a mask • Eye protection • Impervious gown
Transportation and Disposal Procedures	Tips for transportation and disposal procedures include: • Chemotherapeutic agent should be verified between pharmacist and registered nurse. • Disposable instruments and equipment should be used with chemotherapeutic agents to reduce the need of processing instruments that have been exposed to chemotherapeutic agents. • Containers must have a chemotherapy label and should be sent to the sterile processing department. • Chemotherapeutic agents should be transported using a puncture-resistant container before and after the surgical procedure. • Staff must change gloves after chemotherapeutic agent administration and before proceeding with the surgery.
Sterile Processing	Sterile processing department personnel have to wear PPE and must also double-glove when handling and processing chemotherapy contaminated instruments and equipment.

Process	Description
Documentation Protocol for Chemotherapy	The perioperative nurse documents: • Names of the chemotherapeutic agent, medication, dose, route of administration, date, and time of administration • Name of the physician administering the agent • Name of the nurse checking the agent prior to administration
Medication Safety and Chemotherapy Time-Out	Perioperative nurses must monitor patient safety at all times and know what medication and orders the physician has created for the patient. Route of medication administration is especially important in the OR setting.
Acceptable Environment	A designated area should be used for the preparation of chemotherapeutic agents.
Physician Orders	Verbal orders are not acceptable for chemotherapy administration. Orders should be written on a designated chemotherapy order form.

Anesthesia Waste Gases

Anesthesia waste gases refer to potentially noxious fumes that escape when patients are being anesthetized. While a single instance may not be harmful to patients or healthcare providers, constant exposure to low level anesthesia waste gases can result in dizziness, chronic fatigue, headaches, and even cancer. Pregnant female healthcare providers may be vulnerable to miscarriage or harmful, long-term side effects to their fetus; male healthcare providers' sperm may be rendered unviable from prolonged exposure to these gases. While the United States Occupational Health and Safety Administration (OSHA) does not regulate anesthesia waste gases, their website provides guidelines for managing worker exposure. These include regular monitoring of anesthetic equipment for leaks, regularly sampling hospital room air quality, and procedural recommendations for administering anesthesia (such as sealing masks to patients before turning on medical equipment). OSHA also recommends practices such as respirator use.

Blood-Borne Pathogens

Blood-borne pathogens refer to infectious agents found in human blood that can cause infection and also be easily transmitted upon contact. Most healthcare providers are regularly at risk of exposure to blood-borne pathogens, especially if they regularly work with patients' bodily fluids, in operating rooms, or with sharps. OSHA requires that employers of healthcare providers follow its standards for controlling blood-borne pathogen exposure. These standards include implementing a training program to educate employees about the risks and how to mitigate them, protective clothing and equipment requirements, certain preliminary vaccinations before the employee's first day of work, and using sharps-free medical equipment when possible. The most commonly recognized blood-borne pathogens include the hepatitis viruses and human immunodeficiency virus (HIV).

Hands-Free Zone

Hands-free zones are used to minimize risks from sharps handling. Research shows that most sharps injuries occur when healthcare providers are passing them to one another. Hands-free techniques recommend that only one healthcare provider holds a sharp at a time, therefore eliminating passing sharps between two people. Instead, healthcare providers should place a sharp down in a designated area, known as the neutral zone, where the next person can retrieve it. Most healthcare facilities use designated areas in which only a single sharp can be placed, and a standardized verbal hand-off technique to pass the sharp. In addition, some healthcare facilities take hands-free handling one step further by using tools such as forceps to handle any sharp, even to place it in the neutral zone. This practice aims to ensure that a healthcare provider does not ever make actual hand contact with a sharp.

Methyl methacrylate is a liquid used to make plastics. It is commonly seen in healthcare settings, especially in oral and dental surgeries. However, direct contact with this substance can cause both short-term and long-term negative effects. These can include headaches, chest pain, coughing, general respiratory issues, temporary issues in the nervous system, and the potential for fetal abnormalities in pregnant women.

MSDS

A material safety data sheet (MSDS) was regularly found in healthcare facilities, laboratories, and other settings where chemicals are used. It provided information about relevant chemicals, how to store and use them, potential risks, and how to manage hazards that may occur. After 2012, the United States adopted the safety data sheet (SDS) information system, which stems from the Globally Harmonized System of Classification and Labelling of Chemicals. This system is an international standard for chemical safety. It covers 16 comprehensive sections relating to chemical mixtures, identifying hazards, ingredient information, first aid responses to potential hazards, action required in the event of accidental spills, handling and storage, exposure, toxicology, ecological considerations, proper waste management, transportation considerations, and regulatory information as set forth by the country of location.

CJD

Creutzfeldt-Jakob Disease (CJD) is a fatal brain disorder that occurs around age 60 or later. Symptoms include a sudden onset of dementia that rapidly intensifies, loss of muscle coordination and function, loss of mental focus and clarity, loss of vision, and insomnia. Patients eventually go into a coma, which leads to brain death and/or other organ failure. CJD cases can be sporadic, where the case occurs randomly with no risk history in the patient. Hereditary CJD cases can exist but are less common. Acquired CJD occurs as a secondary result of a medical procedure, but this type of CJD is still somewhat mysterious as the disease itself is not infectious. CJD is commonly diagnosed as dementia or meningitis; it often is not recognized as the cause of death until an autopsy is performed. An autopsy usually reveals large holes in the patient's brain where neural tissue has degenerated. There are no known treatments, and researchers are still uncertain what exactly causes CJD. Some researchers believe that it is caused by a blood-borne virus, but there is no scientific evidence for this yet.

Personal Protective Equipment

Personal protective equipment (PPE) refers to any equipment used to protect the wearer from hazardous materials such as bodily fluids, chemicals, radiation, noxious gases, blunt objects, or other entities that could cause personal injury upon contact, consumption, or inhalation. PPE can also be used to protect an individual from loud sounds. PPE can include shoe covers, reinforced types of shoes, hazardous material suits, face masks, respirators, earplugs, earmuffs, bulletproof vests, sturdy materials for daily work clothing, hardhats, helmets, and so on. The United States Occupational Health and Safety Administration (OSHA) is an agency dedicated to ensuring employers in the US maintain high safety standards for its employers. Standards vary by industry. However, OSHA requires that employers train all workers in the safety precautions that pertain to their industry and job role. This includes PPE training and ensuring that issued equipment fits well and is in good condition.

Healthcare providers often work with PPE that protect them from infectious patients. These commonly include items like gloves, surgical masks, surgery gowns and booties, and protective eyewear. Healthcare providers also require PPE that protect them from hazardous material that is not biological in nature, such as medicinal compounds or disinfecting agents, especially if they regularly work in a laboratory setting.

Standard Precautions

Standard precautions are general precautions to be used with all patients in a medical setting. These precautions include personal protection if the patient is suspected to have a contagious disease, environmental cleanliness, disinfection and sterilization of all medical equipment and linens, safe sharps handling, and safe infectious waste disposal techniques. Hand hygiene is one of the most critical precautionary practices. All healthcare providers should wash their hands with soap and water when entering or exiting a patient's room, any time they come into contact with bodily fluids, when removing gloves, before and after touching any medical equipment, before eating, and after using the restroom. In addition to these hand washing guidelines, regular use of alcohol-based hand sanitation throughout the workday is also recommended.

Transmissions-Based Precautions

Transmissions-based precautions are used in addition to standard precautions when the presence of highly infectious patients are suspected. These precautions are implemented even while laboratory testing to confirm an infectious agent is conducted. Though this process can take days or weeks, it is necessary in order to control the spread of the infectious agent. Transmission-based precautions encompass contact, droplet, and airborne precaution guidelines.

Biological and Chemical Monitoring

Biological Indicator

A biological indicator is used as a control system to test if sterilization techniques are working effectively. It is constructed using a square of metal that can withstand the heat requirement within the sterilization technique. The surface area of the metal is marked with resistant bacteria. The metal is then placed inside the sterilizing chamber (such as a steam chamber or autoclave) with the ideal goal of killing all spores on the metal sheet. The metal is placed in an area of the chamber where it is least likely for this goal to be met (such as near the very bottom where the air is coldest, or other areas where manufacturers recommend avoiding placement). After undergoing the sterilization process, the metal is incubated in conditions that would promote bacterial growth.

If there is bacterial growth after the incubation period, the biological indicator does not pass the sterilization test and the technique must be revised. This may require a change in mechanical inputs (such as higher temperatures within the chamber), a procedural fix (such as placing the holding bag only in the upper half of the chamber), an equipment fix (such as addressing a broken part that is preventing the chamber from reaching validated input points), or a massive overhaul of the sterilization technique.

Bowie-Dick Dynamic Air Removal Test

The Bowie-Dick test is performed in dynamic air removal steam sterilization systems. Dynamic air removal systems operate in conjunction with a vacuum mechanism that removes air out of the chamber as steam enters. If the air is not fully removed, steam cannot enter the holding bag that contains the instruments that need sterilization. The Bowie-Dick test runs vacuum suction and steam bursts in intervals with a test load. This checks that both are operating at the pressure needed for the steam to enter the holding bag. If a Bowie-Dick test is successful, the sterilization process will take place with medical equipment in the chamber. Many sterilization facilities run Bowie-Dick tests daily. In a highly standardized facility, failure of this test will be rare and indicate a need for equipment repair.

Chemical Indicator

A chemical indicator shows any changes occurring to chemical or physical properties within a sterilization chamber. It may show changes occurring in surface material, pH, texture, temperature, or some other way that is visible to the eye. These are used to determine if sterilization technique processes are working in the manner for which they are designed. In manufacturing, chemical indicators are used in three contexts.

Class 1 chemical indicators, also known as process indicators, are simple items that show if an item has been exposed to a specific process or not. These can include items such as a sticky seal on a package that would be closed if the package had undergone a sealing process, or open if it had not. Additionally, some Class 1 chemical indicators are able to show whether or not a process is working properly across all steps. For example, bubbling across a sticky seal could indicate that it is not fully closed, even if it otherwise appears to be sealed.

Class 2 chemical indicators are specialized to specific processes. Their use will vary based on the parameters of the process.

Class 3 chemical indicators are measured across a single specific interval, such as time. They usually serve as benchmarks throughout a specific process.

Class 4 chemical indicators include multi-variable parameters, such as measuring an output at specific time and pressure points.

Class 5 chemical indicators, also known as integrating indicators, are able to perform the functionality of a biological indicator as well as specific CI responses to time, pressure, and temperature.

Class 6 chemical indicators, also known as emulating indicators, respond to time, pressure, and temperature but do not work in conjunction with a biological indicator.

Chemical indicators, regardless of level, are valid only immediately upon the completion of the process for which it is being utilized. If the item is not checked immediately, it may need to undergo the entire sterilization process again.

Temperature

Pressure and temperature are two of the three critical mechanical variables (along with time) used in BI and CI monitoring tests. Certain pressure gradients are required in sterilization chambers to allow air to be removed from the chamber in order for steam or some other sterilizing solution to penetrate porous holding bags containing medical equipment. High temperatures heat steam in order to kill bacterial spores, viral strands, or fungal matter. Other sterilizing solutions may or may not need to be heated in order to be effective. If pressure levels, temperature, or timing is slightly off, it can cause the holding bag to melt, deflate, or burst; additionally, low levels can prevent incomplete sterilization from taking place.

Environmental Conditions of Sterilization and Storage Areas

A crucial aspect of any surgical procedure is to maintain the sterility of instruments and equipment. Re-usable surgical instruments must be sterilized after each use. Nurses must be familiar with facility policies on handling and storing sterile items.

After a surgical instrument has been used, it must be decontaminated before it can be sterilized. The area of decontamination may require negative pressure ventilation to prevent airflow into adjacent rooms. Supervisory nurses may be tasked with ensuring that the rooms are set to operate under negative pressure. A commonly used tool to check for negative pressure is the "tissue test," where a piece of tissue is placed on the floor by the door. If the tissue is pulled towards the room, it indicates the room is negatively pressurized. After decontamination, the items are dried and placed in containers for sterilization.

Sterilization is performed under strict, temperature-controlled conditions. Daily monitoring of the cycle time and temperature should be conducted to ensure it meets regulatory guidelines. The results should be appropriately documented according to facility policy. After sterilization, the instruments are wrapped, packaged, and stored.

Storage areas must meet certain guidelines to ensure that the instruments remain sterile. Factors such as personnel traffic, space, storage configuration, ventilation, and personal hygiene must be monitored consistently. Sterile packages should be stored to allow circulation from all angles. Packages should not be stacked on top of each other. The most important environmental factors to consider are humidity, air exchange, and temperature. If the temperature and humidity of the storage room are too high, this can promote bacterial growth. Alternatively, if the temperature and humidity are too low, they can affect the performance of certain instruments and materials. Air exchange and ventilation must be monitored to prevent contaminated airflow between the storage area and other rooms.

Guidelines Regarding Proper Surgical Attire

The use of personal protective equipment (PPE) and surgical attire is dependent on the area of practice. Facility policies on the use of surgical attire and PPE should be based on recommendations from the Centers for Disease Control and Prevention and the Occupational Health and Safety Administration. The surgical zones are divided into restricted, semi-restricted, and non-restricted (or unrestricted) areas.

Non-restricted, or unrestricted areas, are areas where the risk of contamination is low. These areas include the post anesthesia care unit (PACU), holding area, and OR waiting room. Personal hygiene should be maintained, and aseptic practices (such as hand washing) should be followed. Nurses should be mindful of disposing contaminated attire that may have been worn in a restricted area. For example, if the nurse's hair cover became soiled with the patient's bodily fluids during the procedure, the hair cover must be discarded before entering other zones.

Semi-restricted areas are near the operating room and storage rooms for clean or sterile instruments. Personnel traffic in these areas should be kept to a minimum, and PPE is required. The fabric of surgical attire should follow facility policy, be free of lint, and allow for breathability. The Association of Surgical Technologists recommends fabrics made of material such as polypropylene to decrease the amount of skin and lint shedding. Hair covers should be worn, including beard covers if applicable.

Restricted areas include the scrub sinks and procedure rooms. Surgical attire and PPE should be strictly adhered to. In addition to hair covers, disposable shoe covers, masks, and gowns should also be applied. Surgical gowns provide an additional barrier to prevent contamination of high infection risk surgeries, such as joint replacements with implanted hardware.

Practice Quiz

1. What category of disinfectant is peracetic acid?
   a. High level
   b. Moderate level
   c. Intermediate level
   d. Low level

2. Which of the following is an example of a critical item under the Spaulding Classification System?
   a. Bed rails
   b. Implant
   c. Laryngoscope blade
   d. Endoscope

3. A bedpan is an example of what type of item under the Spaulding System?
   a. Critical item
   b. Semicritical item
   c. Baseline critical item
   d. Noncritical item

4. Why should an instrument remain moist during and after the procedure?
   a. Keeping an instrument moist is a requirement for proper disposal.
   b. Keeping an instrument moist prevents biofilm from forming during the procedure.
   c. Keeping an instrument moist is an optional practice and is not a mandatory practice.
   d. Keeping an instrument moist is a precursor to entry into the sterilizer.

5. Who is responsible for administering chemotherapeutic agents in the OR?
   a. Circulating nurse
   b. Scrub nurse
   c. Pharmacist
   d. Surgeon

Answer Explanations

1. A: Peracetic acid is a high-level disinfectant. There are three categories associated with disinfectants: high level, intermediate level, and low level. Each category has different capabilities in which they destroy bacteria, microorganisms, viruses, or fungi. Peracetic acid can be useful in cleaning semicritical items.

2. B: Implant. Critical items are those that enter the vascular system or sterile tissue. They pose the greatest risk of infection for the patient and have a high risk of causing infection.

3. D: A bedpan is an example of a noncritical item. These are devices that do not physically come in contact with mucous membranes.

4. B: Perioperative personnel should keep instruments moist using sterile water to prevent biofilm from forming on instruments that may enable microorganisms to form.

5. D: The nurse will check medication with the pharmacist using standard medication practices; however, the surgeon will administer the chemotherapeutic agent in the operating room.

Emergency Situations

Identifying Emergency Situations

Nurses must always be prepared to encounter emergency situations in the operating room. Emergencies include patient-related occurrences, medication-induced adverse reactions, and environmental disasters.

Patient-related emergencies require a prompt diagnosis and a coordinated response by the surgical team. Some emergencies include a code arrest, anaphylactic reaction, massive hemorrhage, and incorrect surgical procedures. Facilities should be equipped with policies regarding the management of patient-related emergencies. In a code arrest, duties are designated to the different team members to ensure the best patient outcome. During assessment of the operating room, the nurse must ensure that code arrest equipment and medications are available, including a crash cart, respiratory supplies, and emergency medications. Massive hemorrhage can occur during any surgery, and the nurse should anticipate the administration of blood, intravenous fluids, medications, and extra supplies. Incorrect surgical procedures can result in sentinel events and legal concerns. To minimize this type of emergency, the nurse should ensure that universal protocol is performed before the procedure.

One of the most common environmental emergencies in the operating room is a fire. Fire emergencies may involve the patient or the surroundings. Facilities frequently conduct fire drills to ensure that the staff is prepared to react in a timely manner. In the operating room, attempts to extinguish the fire are performed prior to making the decision to evacuate. Some of the factors that contribute to a fire include faulty electrical equipment, alcohol-based skin preparations, and the use of oxygen. It is important to make sure that fire equipment and supplies are available prior to the start of the procedure. These include fire extinguishers, sterile saline for patient involved fires, and backup respiratory supplies. The nurse should also know the location of the gas shut-off valves, which may need to be manipulated to stop the flow of gases into the operating room during a fire.

Malignant Hyperthermia

While **malignant hyperthermia (MH)** is rare, it is a life-threatening disorder that can be chaotic for an unprepared surgical team. Susceptibility to MH is hereditary, and it can be triggered by commonly used succinylcholine and anesthetic gases. Early signs of MH may include jaw clenching, unexplained tachycardia, muscle rigidity, and an increase in EtCO2. If untreated, the patient's core body temperature can rise to a dangerous level. During an MH crisis, immediate, aggressive treatment is essential. Dantrolene is the first line of treatment for MH, and the initial recommended dose is 2.5 mg/kg. Other common drugs used during an MH crisis include insulin in a glucose solution and calcium chloride. Calcium channel blockers should not be used. While MH may be somewhat unpredictable, all of the surgical team should be aware of their roles and responsibilities in an MH crisis to ensure prompt treatment.

It is imperative that patients be screened preoperatively for MH. Patients may not refer to the condition by name, but the circulator should be suspicious if the patient mentions unspecified anesthesia complications from a previous surgical procedure or in their family's surgical history. If MH is suspected, the circulator is responsible for making the surgical team aware of the potential for this emergency and preparing for a potential crisis. The anesthesia team should be notified immediately so that they can prepare the anesthesia machine and drugs appropriately. Emergency equipment and drugs, typically stored on an MH treatment cart, should be readily available. It is recommended that thirty-six vials of dantrolene be available at all times.

In the event of an MH crisis, the circulator should initiate the call for help and request assistance from any available personnel. The anesthesia team will need to focus on the treatment protocol, and the circulator should assist as needed. For example, dantrolene will need to be reconstituted with 60 milliliters of sterile water, and the circulator and other nurses can perform this duty while the anesthesia team concentrates on the patient. A Foley catheter should be placed if not already present. If the patient's core body temperature rises, the circulator (or delegated personnel) may need to provide ice to cool the patient directly and/or chilled IV solutions for infusion, irrigation, and catheter irrigation.

Anaphylaxis

Another rare but dangerous condition that may prevent itself in the operating room (OR) is anaphylaxis. **Anaphylaxis** is a severe allergic reaction that, outside of the OR, typically presents as a rash, swelling of the throat, hypotension, and/or shortness of breath. However, in the OR, detection of anaphylaxis can be difficult because the patient cannot complain about their symptoms and may be covered in drapes. The most common trigger for an anaphylaxis reaction during surgery is exposure to latex. Other triggers include many of the drugs most commonly used in the OR: penicillin, succinylcholine, rocuronium, propofol, isosulfan blue, and iodine contrast dye. Immediate treatment of anaphylaxis is to remove the suspected source, if possible. As the cause may be an administered drug, treatment should focus on Basic Life Support (BLS) protocols, administration of epinephrine, airway management, and fluid administration.

Again, one of the most common causes of anaphylactic reactions during surgery is exposure to natural latex rubber. Patients should be assessed preoperatively for a potential latex allergy. As it can be hereditary, the circulator should ask about the patient's allergies along with any family members' allergies to latex. In particular, if a patient is allergic to bananas, they may also be allergic to latex. When a potential latex allergy is suspected, the circulator is responsible for alerting the surgical team and ensuring the room is prepared appropriately, including using only latex-free supplies and latex-free gloves.

Alert Band

Latex Allergy

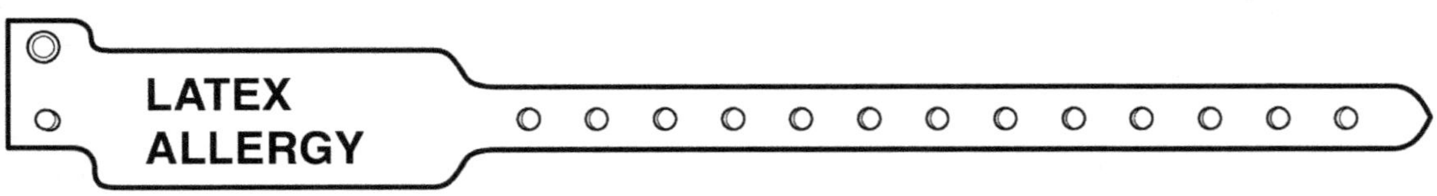

In the event of an anaphylactic reaction, the circulator similarly should initiate the call for help and request assistance from available personnel. Again, the anesthesia team will need to concentrate on prompt treatment, which may include drug and fluid administration. The circulator should assist and delegate as needed.

Cardiovascular Emergencies

Cardiac Arrest

Cardiac arrest can happen to a surgical patient at any time or may be caused by such conditions as malignant hyperthermia or anaphylaxis, as mentioned above. Availability of the "crash cart," or emergency cart, and knowledge of its contents is top priority for all clinical staff in the OR. Any perioperative team member can assist during a "code blue." Generally, the anesthesia staff will be in charge during a code, and the circulating nurse will assist and also delegate duties to other team members.

Advanced Cardiac Life Support

Advanced cardiac life support (**ACLS**) refers to standardized, procedural guidelines to rapidly treat emergency cardiac cases like heart attacks and heart failures, as well as situations that arise from cardiac embolisms, such as strokes. Only certain medical personnel, including registered nurses and nurse practitioners, are allowed to administer the protocols of ACLS. These protocols include analyzing heart rhythms, administering medication intravenously, or performing emergency surgery. Protocols are updated every five years; the most recent version was published in 2015. The 2015 guidelines include using mobile devices to check patient information and contact additional services, limiting chest compression frequency to 120 compressions per minute and chest compression depth to 2.4 inches, pharmaceutical recommendations for drug overdose situations, and separate procedures for cardiac arrests that occur in a medical setting.

Autologous Blood

Autologous blood refers to blood that is collected from a patient in order for reinfusion. The benefits of autologous blood infusion are that it eliminates the potential for infection or rejection, due to the patient's body recognizing the blood as its own. It also prevents accidental infusion of contaminated blood, such as from another patient with a blood disease. Blood may be collected before a patient has a surgery (up to 6 weeks prior), during surgery, or after surgery. The patient may be at risk of anemia or collection and labelling error; autologous blood infusions are also costlier than other forms of blood transfusion.

Blood Loss

Large amounts of blood loss can cause severe complications, including shock, cardiac failure, and/or death. These situations most commonly occur as a result of trauma, illness, or surgical complications. Blood loss can occur through blood leaving the body through an external wound, or it can occur internally. Internal bleeding can quickly become fatal as it is less obvious until symptoms become critical. To treat blood loss, medical professionals can transfuse blood from a safe, compatible source; however, this can cause unwanted side effects such as hemolysis, kidney damage, infection, or allergic reactions if the source of transfused blood is tainted or the wrong blood type for the recipient. If the patient has already progressed to shock or cardiac events as a result of blood loss, they may need to be resuscitated through defibrillation, administered medication, or have fluid imbalances addressed.

Cardiopulmonary Resuscitation

Cardiopulmonary resuscitation (CPR) is a basic life support mechanism administered in emergency situations where a patient is in cardiac or respiratory arrest. CPR can be performed by most people who have been trained in the procedure and does not always need to be administered by a medical professional. In fact, bystanders who capably administer CPR until medical professionals arrive often support a positive recovery outcome for the patient. CPR incorporates chest compressions, conducted by the rescuer who interlaces one hand over the other and places the heel of the bottom palm over the patient's sternum. Compressions should go to a depth of 2.4 inches and occur at a frequency of 100 to 120 compressions per minute. Airway management techniques, such as the head-tilt, chin-lift maneuver or assisted ventilation, should take place along with the compressions. Airway management allows oxygenated air into the body, while compressions help to circulate oxygenated blood.

Circulating Blood Volume

Circulating blood volume refers to how much blood is effectively circulating (through the deoxygenating and oxygenating processes) through a person's body. Adult bodies hold approximately five liters of blood. Expected blood volume is calculated by taking a person's weight in kilograms, multiplying it by 75 milliliters, then multiplying the total by .001 to determine the total number of expected liters of blood. Actual circulating blood volume can be measured through non-invasive testing methods.

Circulation

Circulation refers to the process of moving blood throughout the body, therefore allowing oxygen, hormones, and nutrients to reach the individual cells of organ and tissues. In system circulation, oxygenated blood from the lungs travels to the heart and is pumped to the rest of the body through a network of vessels called arteries. Oxygenated blood travels to muscles, the brain, and all of the visceral organs. Once used, deoxygenated blood travels through vessels called veins back to the heart, which pumps it into the lungs to become oxygenated once more. Lymph, a fluid that supports the body's immune system and cellular waste disposal, also circulates throughout the body and is pumped by the heart.

Deep Vein Thrombosis

Deep vein thrombosis refers to a clot that forms in a deep vein (as opposed to a superficial vein). Deep veins are responsible for critical deoxygenating processes; therefore, clots in these veins can cause serious complications, such as blockages. Deep vein thrombosis is characterized by swelling, pain, and warmth. It most commonly occurs in the lower legs.

Dysrhythmia

Dysrhythmia refers to any abnormal rhythm of the heart muscle. These include forms of tachycardia (a heart rate averaging above 100 beats per minute) and bradycardia (a heart rate averaging below 60 beats per minute). Some dysrhythmias are asymptomatic or temporary (such as an increased heart rate after drinking a caffeinated beverage), while others are critical and must be carefully managed (such as with an implanted pacemaker).

Embolus

An embolus is a mass found in blood vessels. Most often, it is a clot compromised of fatty acids, cholesterol, or blood. However, they also can be bubbles of air or gas. Emboli can block passageways and prevent adequate blood circulation from occurring. Fatty acids, cholesterol, and blood embolisms normally result from the build-up of these substances over time, which then break off and travel through the body's extensive blood vessels until they are snagged by vessel walls or otherwise unable to pass. Air embolisms occur from wounded or punctured vessels, while gas embolisms most commonly occur in deep sea divers who dive or resurface too quickly. In these situations, air pressure imbalances cause gas bubbles inside the divers' blood vessels.

Fluid Replacement

Fluid replacement is the practice of replacing specific fluids that have been lost due to trauma, pathology, environmental factors, or surgical complications. It is most commonly needed in situations of excessive heat, gastrointestinal disease, or malnutrition and dehydration. Fluid can be replaced orally or intravenously. Dehydrated patients often need solutions containing water and an electrolyte mix based on the substances in which the patient is deficient. Comparatively, patients who have lost blood or plasma will need blood transfusions to replace the lost fluid.

Hypertension

Hypertension refers to elevated systolic or diastolic blood pressure. It is generally defined as a systolic reading of 140 or higher, or a diastolic reading of 90 or higher. Prolonged periods of hypertension are considered a critical condition that can potentially lead to seriously adverse outcomes, such as heart attack, aneurysms, stroke, or metabolic disorders. This is due to the constant burden on the walls of the blood vessels that ultimately makes it difficult for blood to circulate adequately.

Hypotension

Hypotension refers to low systolic or diastolic blood pressure. It is generally defined as a systolic reading of 90 or lower, or a diastolic reading of 60 or lower. Some endurance athletes may be prone to hypotension without any serious consequences. Other adults may have chronic hypotension with mild dizziness, but no debilitating symptoms. Elderly patients or patients who are at risk of going into shock are considered critical if they appear hypotensive, as this can indicate that oxygenated blood may not be circulating to crucial organs, such as the brain.

Shock

Shock refers to instances of extremely low blood pressure resulting in inadequate blood circulation. This is considered an emergency situation. Shock can occur from infection, extreme blood loss, spinal cord injury, or a severe allergic response. Patients may appear unresponsive and feel cold to the touch. Based on the type of shock, patients will be treated with fluid replacements, antibiotics, and/or immobilization.

Thrombus

A **thrombus** is a clot of blood. It most commonly occurs in autonomous wound repair to slow bleeding and support wound healing. In pathologic cases, clotting occurs at levels that can cause blockages in blood vessels. Some people, such as those with congenital heart diseases or leukemia, are predisposed to this condition and must be monitored for even minor injuries.

Transfusions

Transfusions refer to replacements of blood, plasma, platelets, lymph, or specific blood cells. Patients may need transfusions in situations of extreme blood loss, in instances of blood disorders, or in instances of blood infections. While safeguards to ensure blood donations are tested for blood type and disease, recipients of transfusions may still experience complications such as hemolytic reactions, allergic reactions, rejection, lung injury, sepsis, or contraction of a disease.

Trauma

Trauma refers to any event that results in lasting physical, physiological, or psychological damage to an individual. This definition encompasses a wide range of events, including, but not limited to, natural disasters, combat service, sexual assault, and incidences of violence against an individual or one that results in mass casualties. Traumatic injuries refer to mild to critical injuries that occur to an individual from an external force. Depending on the severity, traumatic injuries can quickly heal in outpatient settings or may require extensive, long-term care in a medical setting.

ARDS

Acute respiratory distress syndrome (ARDS) is characterized by fluid buildup in the lungs that ultimately leads to loss of respiratory function. It is rarely a primary condition; there is normally an underlying condition that leads to ARDS. These include sepsis, pneumonia, or blunt force injury to the chest, head, or neck. Since many patients are already compromised in some other way, the recovery rate is low. In those patients who do survive, they are likely to experience some degree of permanent lung damage, loss of memory and focus due to periods of inadequate oxygen supply to the brain, and/or depression.

Blunt Trauma

Blunt trauma refers to any bodily injury caused by external force that does not immediately break or penetrate the skin. These can range from mild in severity, such as trauma that results in superficial bruising and heals with minimal medical intervention, to extreme, where vital organs are compromised due to the location and intensity of force. Areas commonly affected by blunt trauma include the head and the abdomen. This type of trauma can occur in motor vehicle accidents, assaults, falls, recreational sports, and disaster contexts. Blunt trauma can result in secondary injuries such as bruising, concussions, lacerations, hemorrhage, organ rupture, and internal injuries. The majority of blunt traumas that require emergency care are investigated for influences such as assault or substance abuse.

DIC

Disseminated intravascular coagulation (DIC) is a rare but serious condition in which blood clotting becomes abnormal and overactive. This leads to the buildup of clots within the body that can cause blood vessel obstructions. In other instances, the clots promote continuous internal bleeding. DIC is commonly seen as a secondary condition in cancer patients, in cases where blood transfusions are rejected by the recipient, in patients with organ infections, in patients with severe tissue injury, and in septic patients. It can come on unexpectedly, and up to 50 percent of patients who experience DIC die. Patients who survive may experience permanent organ damage.

DNR

Do Not Resuscitate (DNR) instructions are legal instructions provided by a patient, the patient's family, or the patient's power of attorney before serious medical procedures in which heart or lung failure could occur. These instructions guide medical providers to allow a natural death rather than repeated attempts at resuscitating a patient. Elderly and immunocompromised patients often have a slim chance of survival in these contexts, and DNR instructions aim to minimize invasive, potentially ineffective, and costly procedures for patients that may not benefit from them.

End of Life Care

End of life care refers to guidelines and procedures to comfort terminal patients. Depending on the patient and the condition, this period may last a few days or can last months. During this time, patients may be moved into a hospice facility, receive comfort measures at home, create any legal documents that support their family members in decision-making (such as advance directives or wills), and receive grief counseling with their loved ones.

Mechanism of Injury

Mechanism of injury is an explanatory term used to detail the sequence of events which caused the occurrence of a traumatic bodily injury. This information can provide insight into the severity of an injury. Examples of mechanisms of injury can include the sequence of events related to a fall (i.e., an elderly patient fell from standing height onto a concrete surface, a construction worker fell from a two-story scaffolding structure onto a grassy hill), a motor vehicle accident (i.e., a car was hit head-on at a speed of 70 miles per hour, a car hit a tree at a speed of 11 miles per hour), a penetrating wound (i.e., a patient received a point-blank gunshot wound from a handgun, a patient stepped barefoot onto a small nail), or any other traumatic injury. However, all mechanism of injury reports should include comprehensive details such as speeds, heights, objects involved, and other factors that could have influenced the injury.

Multisystem Trauma

Multisystem trauma refers to instances where the patient has injuries to more than one bodily system, such as a gunshot victim who received wounds to the chest (affecting the respiratory system) and the head (affecting the neurological system).

Organ Donor

Organ donors refer to patients who have legally declared that they are willing to donate their organs to research or other patients in need in the event of death. This choice is commonly indicated on state driver's license or identification cards. In some instances, patients can choose to donate organs while still living, such as in the event of a voluntary transplant donation or if a patient is in end-of-life care. There are almost no limitations to donating organs, and facilities take care to treat donors' bodies with compassion and respect.

Rapid Sequence

Rapid sequence intubation is an advanced airway management technique for emergency cases. In this procedure, patients are sedated to the point of unconsciousness and intubated with an endotracheal tube. This is most commonly used in critical cases where time is of the essence, such as in anaphylactic patients or those who need ventilation yet are unable to receive it through bag valve mask techniques. Rapid sequence intubation is also utilized in patients who are at risk of aspiration. This technique should not be used in patients who are already unconscious from their injuries.

Hemorrhage

Hemorrhage refers to any instance where extreme blood loss occurs. It can occur anywhere in the body and can refer to both external and internal cases of blood loss. Hemorrhage cases can be categorized into three classes of severity. Class 1 cases are mild and often do not require medical care. Class 2 cases are more moderate, with patients' bodies trying to compensate for the blood loss. These patients will show symptoms of elevated heart rate and pale skin. Class 2 cases are often easily treated through intravenous fluids. Class 3 cases are severe, with patients losing between 30% and 40% of total volume. Patients are likely to experience shock and require blood transfusions. Class 4 cases are the most critical and the most likely to result in death. They include cases where over 40% of total blood volume has been lost; immediate blood transfusions and other medical interventions are usually necessary in these cases.

Local Anesthetic Systemic Toxicity (LAST)

Local anesthetic systemic toxicity (LAST) is a serious complication that can occur after the injection of local anesthetics such as ropivacaine, bupivacaine, and lidocaine, which are used to numb the tissues surrounding the surgical area. Nerve blocks numb the area around the nerves to decrease pain. Local anesthesia is meant to be administered in a precise location. However, if the medication reaches the systemic circulation, the risk of toxicity is increased. Systemic involvement will result in adverse effects, likely observed immediately post injection. Some adverse effects are delayed depending on the patient's weight, medical history, and concentration of the medication.

Mild LAST is characterized by symptoms involving the central nervous system, such as perioral numbness, confusion, dysarthria, tinnitus, and agitation. The patient may also report a metallic taste in the mouth. Signs and symptoms of moderate LAST include dizziness, blurred vision, drowsiness, and headache. The most severe form of LAST involves the cardiovascular system, resulting in cardiac dysrhythmias, hypotension, bradycardia, and respiratory or cardiac arrest.

The first intervention that should occur if the patient is experiencing symptoms of LAST is to stop the local injection. If mild, the central nervous system effects may subside. The nurse should monitor vital signs and ensure that the patient's airway is intact. Oxygen administration may be indicated if the patient's respiratory system is compromised. If the patient experiences a severe reaction, seizure control is indicated. The nurse should anticipate administering medications such as benzodiazepines. Should the patient proceed to respiratory arrest, ventilatory support is needed. The pharmacological management of LAST involves a lipid emulsion. Lipids bind to the molecules of the anesthetic medication, preventing their systemic effects and reversing the toxicity.

Interdisciplinary Team

The surgical team consists of many members with different roles. The circulator is responsible for awareness of their respective scope of practice. While there are tasks that the circulator can delegate to other team members, they must be careful to ensure that the delegated tasks are within their scope of practice. Further, as the patient's advocate, the circulator should speak up if they observe other team members practicing outside of their scope of practice. Each state or facility may have unique policies and procedures that define scope of practice for team members.

The surgeon may be assisted by another surgeon, fellows, residents, students, and/or FAs. However, there are certain tasks that should be performed by the primary surgeon and not one of their designees. For example, after the surgery is finished, the primary surgeon should be the one to speak with the patient's family. The surgical time-out is initiated by the individual performing the procedure; this can be a surgical fellow or resident, as the facility allows. Also, while the surgeon may delegate opening and/or closing to a designee, the circulator should also know at what point the primary surgeon should be scrubbed in, and they should speak up if another team member proceeds without the primary surgeon's knowledge.

Similarly, the anesthesia care of the patient may involve a team of anesthesia providers. The circulator should be cognizant of what responsibilities are within each team member's scope of practice and what activities require supervision for CRNAs, AAs, and students.

The circulator should ensure that any responsibilities are delegated to other team members qualified to perform these tasks. For example, while another circulator or scrub tech is qualified to open items onto the sterile field, a team member without proper training may compromise the integrity of the sterile field.

OR and Resource Management

Managing the OR requires balancing many factors, including equipment, staffing, and surgeon schedules. Running a successful OR starts with planning and resource management, which should ideally be done prior to the day of surgery. The nurse running the OR should review the schedule in advance and confirm that there are no conflicts for materials or equipment and that there is enough staff scheduled to complete all of the day's procedures. Also, the OR manager should always be prepared for unexpected circumstances to occur on the day of surgery.

In reviewing the schedule, the OR manager should take note of what specialized equipment may be needed for the cases. For example, many cases may require a C-arm or microscope, and the facility may have a limited number of these pieces of equipment. In planning the day, the OR manager should ensure that this equipment will be available so that there are no unexpected delays waiting for equipment.

Also, the staff schedule should be compared to the surgical schedule to ensure there is enough staff available to complete all of the scheduled procedures and to allow for emergency procedures that may also need to be performed. Because staff overtime can be costly to the facility, it is ideal that staff be scheduled for all hours where procedures are scheduled to be performed, as opposed to requiring staff to work overtime in order to finish the day's schedule.

Environmental Hazards

Toxic fumes in the OR can be eliminated by using a smoke evacuator during the procedure. Fumes develop when using electrocautery devices and lasers, and the smoke can be toxic to the patient, as well as the surgical staff. Availability of smoke evacuator tubing/suction and use of filtration surgical masks can help reduce the risk of inhaled fumes.

Many of the unique supplies and drugs used in the OR complete the fire triangle (heat, fuel, oxidizer), and the circulator should be aware of the potential for an intraoperative fire. Prior to the procedure, the circulator should assess the fire risk for the patient and procedure and identify ways to potentially reduce this risk. In particular, the circulator should ensure that any alcohol-based prep solutions dry prior to draping the patient because the electrocautery pencil can start a fire. Also, during laparoscopic cases, the circulator should be vigilant for the potential of the light cord to start a fire if left on the drapes. In the event of a fire, the circulator should assist the team in eliminating any causative sources and protecting the patient. If the fire spreads outside of the patient, the circulator should initiate the facility's fire protocol and request assistance.

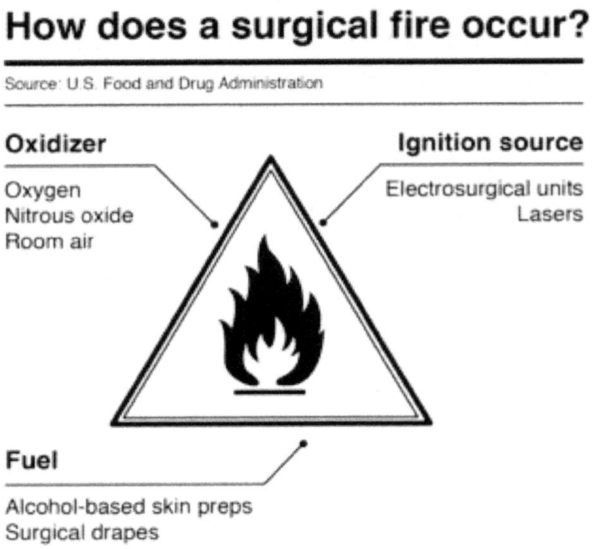

Burn

A burn refers to any instance where tissues of the body are injured from heat, electricity, radiation, cold, friction, or chemicals. Burns are categorized into three types. First-degree burns affect the top layer of skin; they are often mild, may show some redness, and heal well. Second-degree burns affect the superficial layer and deeper layer of the skin. They may be characterized by redness, blistering, and extreme pain. First- and second-degree burns may be treated with cooling liquids, numbing medications, and pain medications. Third-degree burns involve all layers of the skin; they are often painless, as the skin's nerves are usually completely damaged. However, the skin may feel inflexible and smooth to the touch. Functionally, it will be useless; skin grafts may be required. Fourth-degree burns affect the muscles, bone, and fat that are under the skin. Areas of fourth degree burns normally require amputation.

Explosion

Explosions refer to extreme releases of energy, heat, gas, and sound. They can occur naturally or can be manmade. Explosion injuries are often catastrophic or fatal, especially if the explosion occurs in a small space or occurs physically near the victim. Explosions tend to take place most commonly near war or terror sites, in chemical laboratories, or in nuclear plants. Injuries are described in relation to the blast. They are classified in four categories. Primary blast injuries occur from blasts that cause destructive sound waves or high pressure. These tend to destroy organs and other hollow structures that are susceptible to changes in pressure, such as lungs, eardrums, or the stomach. Secondary blast injuries occur from blasts that have debris, such as nail bombs. The more debris and the faster it travels, the higher the injury severity. Tertiary blast injuries occur when a person is physically moved by the force of the blast. Quaternary blast injuries encompass any other injury that doesn't meet the characteristics of primary, secondary, or tertiary injuries.

Fires and explosions can both result in deadly burns, as well as penetrating or blunt force injuries. The extent of damages that both fires and explosions can cause often depend on certain factors. Many explosions automatically result in fires, due to the amount of heat that is generated, the interaction with potential fuel sources, and the presence of oxygen. Fires can make the repercussions of explosions much worse, depending on a few variables: the size of the fire, the source of the explosion (explosions involving combustible chemicals at a chemical plant, for example, may cause more damage than a small, contained explosion in a lab), how flammable the materials around the fire were (as this causes fire to spread more easily), the level of pure, concentrated oxygen that was present (as oxygen causes fires to intensify), and if other fuel sources are available that hinder extinguishing efforts (such as a vehicle explosion, where gasoline is readily present).

Fire Ignition

Fire ignition takes place when the three factors of the "fire triangle" are present. These include heat, a fuel source, and oxygen. Fires can be extinguished when one or more aspects of the triangle are removed. In small fires, the goal is typically to remove the oxygen source. This can be achieved with a standard fire extinguisher, fire blanket, or water. In large fires, such as natural or manmade wildfires that become uncontrollable, firefighters normally focus on eradicating the fuel source. This can be extremely difficult in dry, forest areas where many items are flammable. In these situations, fires can rage on for months and often cause surrounding residential areas to evacuate.

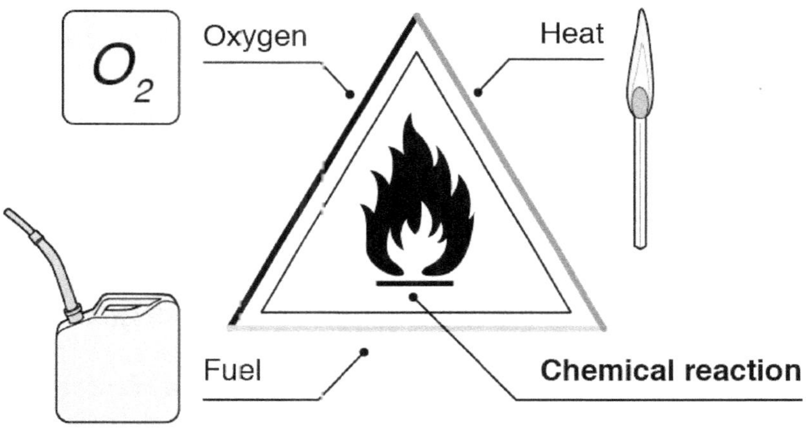

Disasters

Disasters are events where large scales of damage, and often mass injuries and casualties, take place. They are disruptive to communities and can overwhelm the medical facilities in the area. Disasters may be manmade or caused by nature. They often require extended periods of time and resources from outside of the community in order for the area and its citizens to recover.

Bioterrorism

Bioterrorism refers to the use of biological organisms to cause destruction to an individual, group of people, community, or society. Because some pathological organisms, such as smallpox, can be contagious between hosts, a bioterror attack can have widespread consequences and may be difficult to contain. While bioterror attacks have been rare in US history, a spike in events after the World Trade Center attack on September 11th, 2001, have led public health officials to develop health communications on the topic. Initial treatments upon detection are likely to include quarantine and antibiotic use; however, this may not necessarily limit the potential spread of some pathogens.

Bombs

Bombs are explosive devices that can cause destruction, injuries, and death due to extreme shock waves, heat, or projectile matter. Simple bombs are often made of an explosive compound and fuel and cause low pressure changes upon combustion. However, terror attacks have been conducted using simple bombs, made worse by using multiple bombs or filling the bombs with materials that are able to cause penetrating injuries. More serious bombs include those used in wars or large-scale terror attacks. These include highly explosive bombs that result in large shock waves and large changes in pressure, and thermobaric bombs which utilize changes in pressure in addition to extreme heat. Nuclear fusion and fission bombs cause instantaneous death due to high radiation, and are able to destroy entire communities or cities with a single device.

Mass Casualty

Mass casualty incidents refer to manmade or natural disasters that result in the injury or death of multiple victims within a relatively short period of time. These situations are likely to overwhelm trauma, medical, and emergency resources within the affected community. Communities typically have protocols for first responders to follow in the event of a mass casualty incident, and emergency departments of local hospitals will have the same. These protocols may include the establishment of an on-site morgue, specific triage guidelines, and recruiting medical providers and allied health workers from neighboring communities. Depending on the severity of the incident, temporary healthcare facilities and resources may need to be in use for an extended period of time. It is important to note that in mass casualty events, often the healthiest victims arrive at medical facilities first (as they may be able to bring themselves), whereas more severely wounded victims who are in greater need of urgent care arrive later. Hospitals should be equipped with protocols for addressing this situation.

Natural Disasters

Natural disasters refer to destructive events resulting in property and infrastructure damage, injuries to people, animal, and livestock, and ecological devastation. Natural disasters are often mass casualty incidents. They include events such as hurricanes, floods, earthquakes, avalanches, blizzards, landslides, volcanic activity, tornados, heat waves, wildfires, and windstorms. Medical facilities normally have protocols in place to address potential natural disasters that could occur in the surrounding geographic area. These protocols address not only organizational procedures to follow in the event of a natural disaster, but also how to house and/or evacuate victims of specific types of natural disasters. For example, a coastal hospital will likely have procedures in place for hurricanes and flooding, while a hospital near a fault line will likely have procedures in place for an earthquake.

Disaster Preparedness

Disaster preparedness is an important component of the healthcare field as medical providers have an ethical duty to serve during these times. Medical providers should be prepared to work and treat patients not only after mass casualty events, but also during infectious disease crises and mass chemical exposures. These incidents can emerge unexpectedly and last for unpredictable lengths of time. Medical providers must be mindful to not only serve their patients, but to also protect themselves from potentially dangerous situations. This may involve treating patients while using protective barriers, quarantining patients as needed, resting when necessary, and seeking mental health support after crises have passed. Many healthcare providers are susceptible to post-traumatic stress disorders, emotional upheaval, and exhaustion after seeing catastrophic cases and providing the intensive caregiving that is required during disaster events.

Terrorism

Terrorism refers to (often abusive and violent) psychological and physical actions taken by an individual or group to promote fear in another individual or group. These actions are often taken in the name of some ideological cause. Prominent terror attacks that have taken place in the United States include the September 11th attacks in New York City, New York in 2001, a bombing at the Boston Marathon in 2013, and a number of mass shootings in universities, airports, nightclubs, churches, and concert venues. Terror attacks in recent decades have resulted in mass casualty incidents. Consequently, medical professionals must be well-versed in protocols for terrorist attacks, including how to protect oneself during a potential attack as medical facilities can become targets.

Practice Quiz

1. Which of the following symptoms is NOT an early sign of malignant hyperthermia (MH)?
    a. Tachycardia
    b. Increased temperature
    c. Increased EtCO2
    d. Muscle rigidity

2. In the event of an MH crisis, the circulator should be prepared to perform which of the following actions?
    a. Administer a calcium channel blocker.
    b. Irrigate the open wound with a warm saline solution.
    c. Irrigate the bladder with a cold solution.
    d. Turn off the gas supply to the OR.

3. The circulator is prepared for a severe allergic reaction or anaphylaxis during the procedure. Which medication is most likely involved?
    a. Isosulfan blue
    b. Protamine
    c. Insulin
    d. Dantrolene

4. When the circulator interviews the patient preoperatively, which finding should cause concern for case preparation?
    a. Patient's mother suffers from dementia.
    b. Patient has type 1 diabetes.
    c. Patient takes a beta-blocker regularly.
    d. Patient reports an allergy to bananas.

5. Which of the following would be unlikely to contribute to a surgical fire?
    a. Smoke evacuator
    b. Room air
    c. Laser
    d. Alcohol-based prep

See answers on next page.

Answer Explanations

1. B: Despite the name of the condition, a rise in core body temperature is one of the later signs of MH. Early signs include jaw clenching, unexplained tachycardia, muscle rigidity, and an increase in EtCO2.

2. C: If MH progresses to an increased core body temperature, the circulator should be prepared to insert a Foley catheter, if not already present, and irrigate using a cold solution. If the open wound is irrigated as part of the treatment, it should be with a cold solution. Calcium channel blockers are contraindicated in the treatment of MH. The gas supply does not need to be turned off when treating MH.

3. A: Isosulfan blue, which is typically used during sentinel lymph node mapping, is associated with severe allergic reactions. Protamine, insulin, and dantrolene do not require additional vigilance for potential anaphylaxis.

4. D: If the patient reports an allergy to bananas, they may have an unknown allergy to latex. The circulator should ensure that only latex-free gloves and materials are used to set up the case. The other findings do not require adjustments to case preparation.

5. A: It is unlikely that a smoke evacuator would contribute to a surgical fire. The fire triangle consists of three components: an oxidizer, an ignition source, and fuel. Room air contains the oxidizer, oxygen. A laser is a potential ignition source. An alcohol-based prep is a fuel source for an intraoperative fire, and the circulator must ensure it dries before applying drapes.

Professional Accountabilities

Scope of Practice

Perioperative nurses have a number of responsibilities before, during, and after surgery. All perioperative nurses should be aware of what activities are within and outside their **scope of practice**, dependent on their role. There are also different scopes of practices depending on the nurse's role and certification. For example, the scope of practice for a scrub nurse for a procedure will differ from the scope of practice for an RNFA for a procedure. In order to provide the best and safest care, all team members are required to practice within their scope.

Further, the nurse's scope of practice may differ from one perioperative care area to another. While in the preoperative or postoperative phase, administering medications may be a nursing responsibility; however, in the intraoperative phase, this may be an anesthesia responsibility. Nurses should follow the facility's policies and procedures to ensure they are performing duties relevant to the care area and within their scope of practice.

Nurses who serve as managers or in other administrative roles are also bound by the perioperative nursing scope of practice. These roles require coordination and collaboration with other specialties, such as surgeons and anesthesia. When in these roles, the nurse should be aware of the limitations of their scope of practice regarding making medical decisions. In some situations, it may be most appropriate to defer to the surgeon or anesthesia provider for guidance. If there is ever a situation where the nurse questions the judgment of another team member, this concern should be voiced. However, the respective scope of practice in making medical decisions may impact the decision making.

Personal Limitations and Seeking Assistance

Working in the perioperative environment can be stressful, overwhelming, and physically demanding. The day-to-day activities involve more physical activity than in other care areas, especially if the nurse is scrubbed in for the procedure. On top of that, staff members are frequently on call and working overtime. The perioperative nurse is only able to provide the best patient care when they have also taken care of themselves. It is important to remain aware of physical, mental, and emotional health.

The nurse should be aware of personal limitations, physically and mentally, and be cognizant of responsibilities that may put the nurse at risk. Of note, the physical demands of the job can be taxing because many times the perioperative team is positioning or moving an unconscious patient. Whenever needed, the nurse should seek assistance.

Behaviors that Undermine a Culture of Safety

The OR is a unique environment. In this care setting, the mood may be a bit more relaxed after the patient is under anesthesia. However, the team is still required to foster a culture of safe patient care. If a member of the team feels that another team member's behavior, language, or actions undermine or violate the culture of safety, they should be empowered to speak up and voice their concern.

One of the main causes of tension in the OR is related to the proximity of team members in different specialties. It is one of the only areas where the nursing team and two physician-led teams perform their most critical tasks in a single room. At times, there can be "head-butting" or ego-related issues. In order to provide the best care for the patient, the nursing staff should express concern if any other team member's behavior is not contributing to the best case for the patient. In some cases, it may be more appropriate for the perioperative nurse to escalate their concern to their manager to avoid unnecessary tension or arguing in the OR during a procedure, which may negatively impact patient care.

Ethical and Professional Standards

To maintain professional accountability, the circulator should be aware of regulatory standards and guidelines and be cognizant of any changes that may impact their responsibilities or scope of practice. The AORN Standards are one of the most common regulatory standards for the circulator. Regulatory standards exist in order to provide education and updates to best nursing practices.

As a whole, all perioperative nurses should be familiar with the standards and guidelines from OSHA, the ANA, and their respective state. Nurses in all care areas are accountable to these standards.

One of the most helpful guidelines for perioperative nurses are the AORN Standards because they are tailored for the unique environment of the OR and the unique responsibilities of circulators and scrub nurses. The current AORN Standards focus on four domains of patient-centered care: patient safety, patient's physiologic responses to surgical procedures, patient and family behavioral responses to surgical procedures, and the health system where surgery is performed. This model focuses on patient outcomes in each domain. AORN provides a number of standards for perioperative processes and measures for the circulator to abide by.

Another great resource for perioperative nurses is the Perioperative Explications for the ANA Code of Ethics for Nurses. Most nurses are familiar with the ANA Code of Ethics, but this document contains additional information and examples from AORN specific to the perioperative area.

Specific nursing responsibilities and the scope of practice are set forth by the state board of nursing in which the nurse practices. Legal parameters are also defined by each individual state. State boards are also tasked with issuing, renewing, or revoking nursing licenses. Although the nursing scope of practice is similar for every state, nurses must be familiar with the licensing requirements of their individual State Nurse Practice Act. For example, a registered nurse first assistant in the operating room may be required to have a certification in perioperative nursing in the state of Florida, whereas training and experience may be the only requirements in Texas.

Resources for Professional Growth

Perioperative nurses should always be looking for professional growth opportunities. There are varied opportunities both within the facility where the perioperative nurse is currently working as well as outside in other settings. It is sometimes difficult for nurses to consider roles that do not involve direct patient care, but perioperative nurses should try to be open-minded to opportunities that may indirectly improve patient care and the surgery experience.

One option for professional growth that may be available is as a service line manager. For example, a facility may have a nurse manager responsible for the cardiac surgery team or orthopedic surgery team because these specialties may require additional expertise for planning and day-of-surgery operations. Another opportunity may be as the OR charge nurse or manager. While these roles typically involve less direct patient care, they are still incredibly important to successfully running the OR, which impacts the overall patient experience.

Given the wide adoption of electronic medical records, there are also a number of opportunities in information technology (IT) and analytics. This is an exciting area where the perioperative nurse's clinical expertise is invaluable. Within the facility, there may be opportunities to join the IT team to assist with data analysis or system implementation and training. Outside the four walls of the hospital, there are also many opportunities in the vendor community to contribute to design and innovation of products that may be used in the OR. Many of the top health care IT vendors employ perioperative nurses to provide ideas and feedback on how their products may be used in the OR.

Competency

All perioperative nurses should be competent in their practice. While the first step may be awareness of regulatory standards and guidelines, these must be applied to nursing practice in order to be relevant. Each facility may have its own methods for determining and verifying competency in perioperative nursing practice. These may include required hands-on training or web module training and testing.

Continuing Education

Continuing education refers to a range of activities that serve as post-graduate learning. These can be formal activities, such as coursework at an accredited university. Formal activities can also include online courses, seminars, workshops, conferences, and trainings that are relevant to one's field. Participants are often able to earn and document continuing education credits for formal continuing education activities; many fields and certifications require obtaining a certain number of continuing education credits over a period of time during one's career. Continuing education can also take place informally, such as through mentoring from someone who is further along their career trajectory or reviewing new literature that is relevant to one's field.

Lifelong Learning

Lifelong learning is a necessary skill and interest for workers in today's rapidly advancing workforce. As technological and information advances continuously change the landscape of an industry, workers should expect and desire to continuously learn new information in order to remain competent in their fields. Lifelong learning can also promote a tremendous sense of personal growth and accomplishment, build friendships with colleagues, and lead to professional rewards, such as promotions. Medical professionals should strive to not only learn the advances in their fields, but to also self-reflect on the ways they learn best in order to make ongoing education a regular part of their careers.

Professional Organization

Professional organizations are industry-specific groups that serve as a resource for gaining new knowledge, sharing knowledge with colleagues, networking, and skill-building. Professional organizations serve to advance the opportunities and reputation of a specific industry and highlight the ways in which the industry adds value to a community. They may also be responsible for establishing best practices and ethical standards in the field and certifying workers to uphold these principles. When choosing professional organizations for membership, candidates should consider the organization's reputation, membership fees and requirements, and added professional and personal value.

Self-Assessment

Medical professionals should continuously conduct self-assessments of their professional goals, professional interests, and career journey to reflect on achievements they are proud of and determine opportunities for growth. Self-assessments can be guided by online questionnaires designed for this purpose, performance reviews from a close colleague or supervisor, and introspective activities such as journaling. In addition, mapping out goals can highlight the best steps for achieving them. For example, if a registered nurse wanted to move into a management role, he or she may examine what skills and credentials are needed to move into this position. These may prove to be individual opportunities for the registered nurse to pursue.

Quality Improvement Activities

The perioperative nursing team should participate in, and initiate, quality improvement activities in an effort to improve patient care and the overall profession. There are constant opportunities for practice improvement, and ideally, the team should foster an environment that is open to exploring these opportunities.

One of the best opportunities to learn about quality improvement activities is at trade shows and poster presentations. It is very beneficial to review what other institutions have researched or implemented in order to improve patient safety and patient care. These projects can range from changes to workflow and process to introducing tools to improve the hand-off of care in between care areas. After learning about these projects, the perioperative team can determine if implementing a similar project may be beneficial at their own facility while ensuring there are not overwhelming changes that may be a distraction to the team.

With the adoption of electronic medical records and electronic documentation, another great opportunity for research and improvement is using analytic tools to analyze and interpret the data at the facility. There are many examples of perioperative teams using their own data for initiatives such as decreasing turnover times, decreasing postoperative nausea and vomiting (PONV) using premedication, or decreasing unnecessary overtime.

Audit

An **audit** is an inspection of a specific aspect of an organization. Audits can be conducted on procedures, finances, incentives, product counts, or any other area of the business that can be monitored. Audits may be conducted internally or by an external, independent body; most effective organizations perform both types regularly. Audit activities may include checklists of certain processes that must be in place, benchmark score comparisons, and evaluation practices. Internal audits allow organizations to be prepared for external audits. Non-compliance of standards found by an external auditing body, especially if it is regulatory agency, may result in fines, disciplinary action, intensive monitoring, or a shutdown of the organization.

Best Practice

Best practices refer to a set of procedures that are generally accepted to be the most effective method of accomplishing a specific goal. These are shaped by evidence-based practice, professional expertise, and patient or client input. Organizations should follow established best practices in an industry in order to maintain high-quality standards. If an organization is underperforming in an area, researching established best practices for that area and implementing change to reflect best practices is likely to result in improved quality.

Information Literacy

Information literacy is a term used to describe one's research and information gathering skills. This is a relatively new term that resulted from the creation and storage of new information in recent decades. Information literacy is conducive to understanding when information is needed as well as knowing how to procure high-quality, validated, and true information to fulfill a need. This may involve knowing how to perform gap analyses, using technical skills to find information online, and knowing the aspects of scientifically sound research design and significant research findings. Comprehensive information literacy then encompasses the ability to take validated research and information and apply it in a way that solves problems.

Measures

Quality measures are used to determine how effective a quality process is. These can be classified into three categories: structural, process, and outcome measures. Structural measures refer to tools available within an organization that support high quality processes, such as software or highly credentialed personnel. Process measures refer to the assessment of actual steps in a procedure, such as determining if nurses are verifying identity before administering a medical procedure. Outcome measures refer to whether structures or processes in place make a difference, such as number of patients with bedsores in inpatient settings.

Performance Improvement

Performance improvement refers to the process of examining a process or outcome measure, identifying a potential enhancement to the associated process steps, implementing a change to enhance the process, and examining whether any improvements are made in terms of process efficiency or outcomes.

Plan-Do-Study-Act

The **Plan-Do-Study-Act** (PDSA) cycle refers to a framework used to plan and implement tests of change to a process. In the Plan stage, the potential change is documented in great detail. This should include factors such as people involved, resources needed, the actual steps of the new process, and outcomes desired. The Plan stage may include using Lean Six Sigma tools such as process mapping, value stream mapping, and root cause analysis. In the Do stage, the change should be implemented for a predetermined period of time. In this stage, all observations of the workflow and data related to the outcome should be documented. In the Study stage, collected observations and data should be examined to see if they support the desired outcome. In the Act stage, participants should determine whether the change should be kept in place, or if revisions should be made to the new process. There are a number of free PDSA worksheets online that can be used to guide this process.

Quality Assurance

Quality assurance refers to an established system within an organization that has the function of ensuring that processes and outcomes are free of error. Quality assurance practices use administrative and process controls to ensure that variation from the start of the process to the end of the process are limited, therefore creating relatively standardized inputs that lead to an expected output. These factors are associated with efficiency, cost and resource reduction, and reduced product and service defects. Examples of quality assurance practices in the healthcare setting include electronic medical records, which reduce documentation error within and between different healthcare facilities, sanitation checklists, standardized training protocols for staff, and identity verification before medical procedures.

Quality Improvement

Quality improvement is a framework that analyzes performance on a continuous basis to ensure all steps are as efficient and effective as possible. This concept came from manufacturing, where industries focused on reducing defects in product, reducing cost and waste, and worker safety. From a healthcare perspective, quality improvement focuses on patient safety and satisfaction, decreased mortality and medical complications, and personnel job satisfaction. Effective quality improvement in healthcare requires meaningful data, clean and relevant data collection, managing processes of care rather than micromanaging people, and empowering clinicians to take responsibility for quality factors.

Interdisciplinary Teams and Professional Organizations

Accrediting Agency

An **accrediting agency** is a public or private entity that certifies an individual organization as upholding a specific set of competencies or standards. Accrediting agencies may serve internationally, nationally, regionally, state-wide, or locally; they may also be specific to industries. Before pursuing or accepting accreditation from an agency, organizations should ensure that the agency is reputable, high-quality, and provides accreditation that is accepted by and useful to their industry. The Joint Commission is an independent, non-profit accrediting agency that certifies most healthcare organizations (such as hospitals, laboratories, home health services, and so on) for excellence in safety, quality, and patience service.

Best Practice

Best practices refer to a set of procedures that are generally accepted to be the most effective method of accomplishing a specific goal. They often become industry standards to which organizations should aspire and adhere. Best practices are often established through research, clinical expertise, and testing within a specific context. Accrediting agencies may establish best practices from which to audit organizations that are seeking certification. Different industries and different functions will all have different sets of best practices. Organizations may also set forth internal best practices based on industry-wide guidelines, in order to best support their specific goals and outcomes.

Board of Nursing

Each state and territory in the United States has a Nurse Practice Act, under which a **board of nursing** must be established. This board regulates nursing standards, credentials, education requirements, best practices, and licensure within the state or territory. Each area's board of nursing ensures that once standards for licensure are met, they are meticulously maintained throughout one's nursing career in order to uphold high safety and quality standards. If a nurse fails to maintain standards established by their area's board of nursing, they may lose licensure or undergo other disciplinary and corrective actions. If nurses choose to move jurisdictions, they may need to pass requirements for the new jurisdiction. Nurse practice acts and boards of nursing are in place in order to ensure that all forms of nursing, which can take place in a range of settings and with a wide demographic of patients, exhibit competence, skill, quality, and care in all contexts.

Community Standard

Community standards relate to the type of nursing provided. Nurses can work in a range of fields, including hospitals, public health settings, in-home, medical offices, mobile clinics, social programs, and so on. Depending on the type of setting they are in, nurses may provide clinical expertise, nutrition counseling, healthcare administration support, individualized health coaching, clinical monitoring, and other caregiving activities. Therefore, they must be aware of the standards relating to the specific scope of work in which they are practicing.

Evidence-Based Practice

Evidence-based practice employs peer-reviewed systematic research, clinical expertise, and patient desire and value to provide the most comprehensive and holistic intervention for a medical case. There are six main steps to developing an evidence-based resolution in healthcare. These are summarized as Assess, Ask, Acquire, Appraise, Apply, and Self-Evaluate. First, the patient must be assessed. This includes not only conducting a physical, clinical assessment of patients, but also encouraging their involvement by inquiring about specific concerns, ideas, and values toward their health. Second, questions relating to the potential clinical case should be asked. Third, evidence that may support a resolution should be acquired. This may include conducting reviews of scholarly research and soliciting the input of colleagues and mentors. Fourth, review evidence to ensure it is valid and useful. Fifth, all compiled evidence should be shared with the patient and patient input should be solicited again. Finally, the last step should involve self-reflection on behalf of the provider and an assessment from the patient to ensure that useful, valuable, and high-quality care was provided.

Nurse Practice Act

Nursing guidelines are developed in order to provide decision-making advice as it relates to clinical cases. Their goal is to standardize care by utilizing evidence-based practice, provide documented accountability standards for nursing professionals, and generally guide nursing care. Nursing guidelines may be developed nationally, regionally, or within a specific organization. Guidelines are typically developed by reviewing appropriate and relevant scholarly literature, proposing guidelines based on research and the input of key stakeholders, and testing proposed guidelines in clinical settings to determine what aspects work well and consistently and what aspects need further development. Finally, once guidelines are accepted, they should be continuously reviewed and revised as needed in order to maintain high safety, quality, and efficiency standards while incorporating advances in technology or shifts in the healthcare culture.

Position Statement

Position statements are made by a professional organization to explain why the industry promotes a certain course of action. They often incorporate the viewpoints of many professionals in the industry and are valid for certain periods of times. They are often in response to current or emerging news, controversial topics, or emerging trends. For example, the American Nursing Association publicly provides position statements on a number of topics such as infectious diseases, substance abuse, human rights topics, and workplace health.

Recommended Practices

Recommended practices are developed based on evidence-based research and are normally approved by a governing body of the field. For example, the Association of perioperative Registered Nurses (AORN) recommends best practices for perioperative nursing procedures. Recommended practices are developed and shared in order to proactively address potential issues, concerns, and hazards.

Regulation

Regulations are established for an industry by bodies of authority, such as the government or independent agencies. They are established in order to ensure certain functions take place in a particular way in order to reach a specific outcome.

Standard

Standards for the nursing profession allow the comparison of actual practice to compare to best practices. Standards guide operating procedures within organizations that employ nurses, serve as performance standards for reviews, and allow management to divide responsibilities based on the credentials each nurse has. Nursing standards can vary based on the level of skill and competency each nurse has acquired, licensure, and personal expertise.

Statute

Statutes are documented legislation created by legal authorities. They are used to govern, create and implement policies, or set rules for specific situations. They may be established at the federal, state, or local level.

Shared Governance

Shared governance is a theoretical model used in the nursing profession to promote high quality care and a healthy work environment. Shared governance combines the inputs and skills of both superiors and subordinate staff to hold nursing professionals accountable for their work. This model also aims to nurture collaborative efforts to providing care that is safe, effective, and considered valuable by the patients. It promotes high levels of cooperation and aims to foster respect between all employees in a hierarchical structure, believing that this leads to improved worker productivity and satisfaction, and consequently, better service delivery. Ways to implement shared governance in a medical setting include defining collaborative efforts and boundaries between different professional roles, soliciting input from all staff members, regular in-person meetings where all members feel comfortable sharing opinions, ideas, and concerns, and reliable modes of communication outside of meetings. Shared governance is associated with stronger feelings of responsibility, group collaboration, and professional support in the work setting.

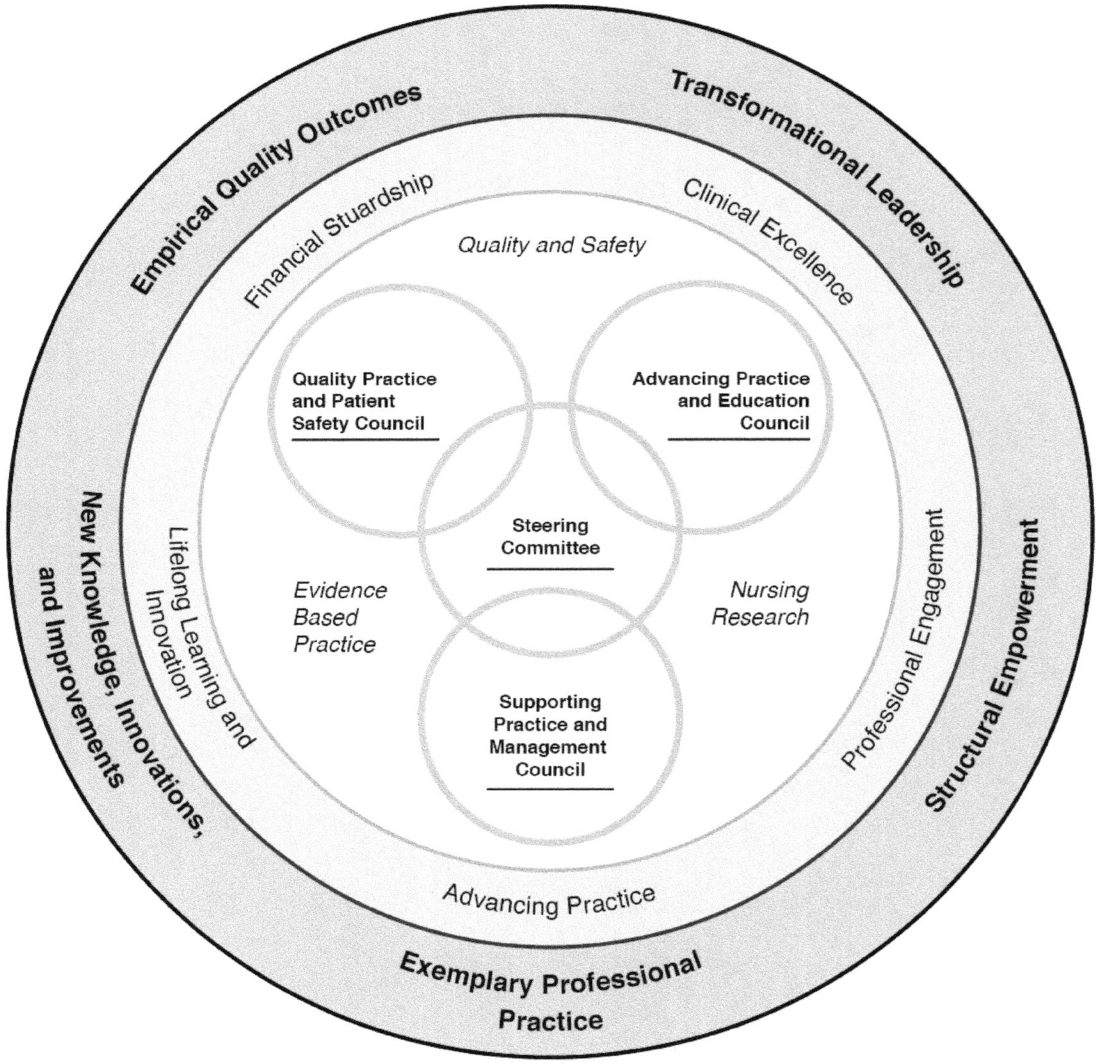

Professional Behavior

Professional Development Activities

In an effort to continually improve and grow as professionals, perioperative nurses are encouraged to participate in professional development activities. Some of these opportunities may be local to the facility where the nurse is employed, such as participating in committees or assisting with staff education. Committees have a wide range, from social and team-building activities to research and process improvement.

Outside of the nurse's place of employment, there are opportunities for advanced degrees and certifications, such as CNOR certification. And nurses who are interested in more involvement as scrubbed personnel may be interested in exploring RNFA certification and careers.

Further, there may be opportunities with organizations such as AORN to participate in committees and governing bodies. This is a great way to stay informed of potential changes to best practices and voice concern.

Chain of Command

In a professional organization, a chain of command refers to a hierarchy of authority in the organizational structure. This often establishes decision-making power, management, reporting relationships, and specific job duties. The goal of a chain of command structure is to provide clarity about roles within an organization, streamline processes, and provide authority and clarity to organizational decisions. In large corporate organizations, a chain of command diagram tends to take on a triangle shape in order to illustrate a distinct top position, clear middle management, and non-management employees as the foundation. In smaller businesses comprised of more lateral colleagues, the chain of command chart may appear more rectangular.

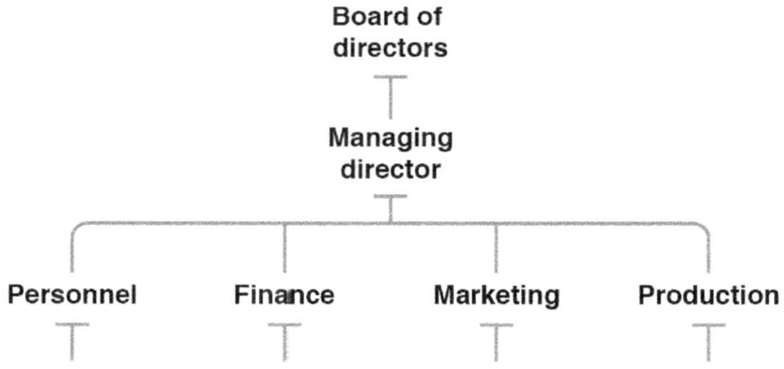

Collegiality

Collegiality refers to the interactions, behaviors, and relationships between colleagues within a single organization or industry. It is typically used to define the actions of individuals with similar skillsets working towards a specific goal. Collegiality is a defining part of an organization's culture, with leadership defining and guiding how relationships between employees are shaped.

Healthy Work Environment

A healthy work environment promotes the safety and job satisfaction of its workers. It supports workers who want to develop professionally and personally, provides a sense of pride and community, is respectful and fair to all workers, and is conducive to workers achieving their defined job responsibilities. Some indicators of a healthy work environment include positive, respectful relationships between all levels of the chain of command, a safe working environment where workers do not feel physically or psychologically threated by internal or external forces, respect for workers' need for work-life satisfaction, fair wages and working hours, and availability of resources for workers to perform their jobs well. Indicators of an unhealthy work environment include workers who feel bullied or harassed, unfair wages and hours, exhausted staff members, high turnover rates, and lack of documented safety standards.

Horizontal and Lateral Violence

Horizontal and lateral violence refers to aggressive behavior toward colleagues that is intended to exhibit displays of power, superiority, and exclusion. It may appear as subtle harassment, bullying, favoritism, physical aggression, or an unjust work environment. Instances of horizontal and lateral violence often leads to other groups of colleagues, or a single individual feeling submissive, helpless, or targeted. This can ultimately lead to feelings of despair, depression, low self-esteem, and lack of professional confidence. Unfortunately, instances of horizontal and lateral violence are well documented in healthcare and nursing professions. Nurses may be subject to hostility from physicians who believe nursing skills are inferior to medicine skills; other nurses who may feel competitive or insecure; and patients who are angry, hurt, or distressed. Encouraging colleagues to work together, to support one another, to empower one another, and to refuse to accept abusive behavior is one way to shift workplace culture away from allowing horizontal and lateral acts of violence to exist. This type of change must often begin from top-down leadership initiatives.

Practice Quiz

1. What should patient tracking boards in the waiting room NOT contain?
    a. The OR number where the case is being performed
    b. The patient's name
    c. The scheduled procedure time
    d. The current status of the case

2. When can details about a case or patient be disclosed?
    a. In the break room where only staff are present
    b. During turnover when preparing for the next case with the turnover staff
    c. Only on a minimum necessary basis
    d. In the cafeteria

3. Which of the following statements is true if the circulator has access to an electronic medical record system?
    a. They have the right to access information on any patient in the system.
    b. They have the right to access information on any patient scheduled for surgery that day.
    c. They have the right to access information on any patient that they have previously cared for.
    d. They have the right to access information on any patient they are currently caring for or preparing for.

4. Which personnel should the circulator rely on to confirm the paperwork associated with blood products?
    a. A CRNA
    b. A radiology technician
    c. The scrubbed personnel
    d. The surgeon

5. After the case, the circulator has paged overhead for moving assistance to help move a heavy patient from the OR table to the transport stretcher. After a few minutes, no personnel have arrived. Which of the following actions is most appropriate?
    a. Attempt to move the patient without additional help.
    b. Ask the circulator who is in an active case next door to help with moving assistance.
    c. Ask the PACU nurse to come to the OR to help with moving assistance.
    d. Wait for the appropriate ancillary team members to be available to help move the patient.

See answers on next page.

Answer Explanations

1. B: In order to protect patient confidentiality, the tracking boards in the waiting room should not contain the patient's name. The OR number, scheduled procedure time, and case status are not elements of PHI, making Choices *A*, *C*, and *D* incorrect.

2. C: Details about a case or patient should only be disclosed when necessary and with the minimum number of people. It is not appropriate to share these details with other staff members unless there is a necessary reason to share this information, making Choices *A* and *B* incorrect. The staff should ensure that in public areas, such as the cafeteria, PHI is not shared, making Choice *D* incorrect.

3. D: With access to an electronic medical record system, the circulator has the ability to access information on any patient in the system. However, this does not give them the right to access information on any patient. The circulator should only access information on their current patient or the next patient scheduled for surgery. They should only access the minimum necessary data.

4. A: CRNA. When confirming blood product paperwork, such as the expiration date/time, the circulator can confirm this with a team member where this activity is within their respective scope of practice. CRNAs, MDs, and other RNs may perform this activity. This activity is outside the scope of practice for radiology technicians and scrub technicians, making Choices *B* and *C* incorrect. The surgeon should not be asked to confirm blood products during the case, making Choice *D* incorrect.

5. D: Wait for the appropriate ancillary team members to be available to help move the patient. The circulator should never attempt to perform an activity that is outside of their personal or physical limitations. If additional help is needed to move or transport a heavy patient, the team should wait until this help is available, even if it delays transportation to PACU.

Practice Test

Pre/Postoperative Patient Assessment and Diagnosis

1. Which statement is accurate regarding preoperative diagnostic procedures?
   a. Diagnostic procedures are only performed the day before surgery.
   b. The hospital setting is most appropriate for performing diagnostic procedures.
   c. The diagnostic procedures performed depend on the planned surgical procedure, patient's history, best practice standards, and risk factors.
   d. The diagnostic procedures ordered are always based on the type of surgery scheduled.

2. In reviewing the patient's preoperative orders, the nurse discovers the preoperative cardiac catheterization has not been done. Which of the following is an appropriate nursing intervention related to diagnostic testing?
   a. Ask the patient why they didn't schedule the cardiac catheterization prior to the day of surgery.
   b. Allow the patient to eat breakfast because the surgery will be canceled.
   c. Proceed with preparing the patient for surgery. Since the patient has been free of chest pain for six months, the surgeon and anesthesiologist are probably OK without seeing the cardiac catheterization report.
   d. Notify the surgeon and anesthesiologist of the missing cardiac catheterization report.

3. Which assessment technique would the nurse employ to obtain subjective data?
   a. Auscultation
   b. Palpation
   c. Percussion
   d. Patient interview

4. How are screening tools used in the preoperative assessment?
   a. They show abnormal lab values
   b. They reveal risk factors that warrant a focused plan of care.
   c. Screening tools decrease the likelihood of using interdisciplinary teams in the plan of care.
   d. The use of screening tools is not recommended in the preoperative phase.

Use the following scenario to answer questions 5–6.

Mrs. Johnson is a 32-year-old patient with newly diagnosed lymphoma. She is tearful during the preoperative interview. She has been married for twelve years and has three young children. In addition to working part time, she is actively involved in church and enjoys volunteering with her children's school activities. She is scheduled to have a cervical mediastinal exploration with lymph node biopsy today for staging of lymphoma. Chemotherapy begins this week.

5. Which NANDA-approved nursing diagnosis is most applicable to Mrs. Johnson's situation?
   a. Anxiety related to the disease process
   b. Risk of hypothermia related to the surgical process
   c. Dehydration related to NPO status
   d. Impaired skin integrity related to prolonged surgical procedure

6. In what phase of care does the nurse begin implementing interventions based on Mrs. Johnson's plan of care?
   a. At six-week follow-up visit
   b. Intraoperative
   c. Preoperative
   d. Postoperative

7. In the patient identity phase of Universal Protocol, the nurse uses which two identifiers?
   a. Name and social security number
   b. Social security number and verification of surgical site
   c. Name and date of birth
   d. Name and verification of surgical site

8. Which statement is true about surgical site marking?
   a. The surgical site should be marked with an "X."
   b. The patient should be involved in the surgical marking process, when possible.
   c. The surgeon should avoid marking the surgical site with "yes" or with the surgeon's initials.
   d. Surgical site marking should not be visible after surgical draping is completed.

9. In which situation should surgical consent be obtained from the patient's power of attorney (POA)?
   a. The patient is twenty years old.
   b. The patient displays a flat affect.
   c. The patient took narcotic medication yesterday.
   d. The patient has Alzheimer's dementia and is oriented to name only.

10. Consent is not required in which situation?
   a. Pediatric procedure
   b. Invasive procedure
   c. Routine procedure
   d. Emergent procedure

11. Advance directives address the patient's wishes in regard to what?
   a. Religious support
   b. Culturally based care
   c. Do not resuscitate (DNR) status
   d. Postoperative pain management

12. The information in the patient's Advance Directives should be shared with which surgical team member(s)?
   a. Surgeon and surgical technologist
   b. Anesthesiologist and circulating nurse
   c. Surgeon and circulating nurse
   d. The entire surgical team

13. Gathering objective data such as vital signs and laboratory values occurs during which step of the nursing process?
    a. Implementation
    b. Assessment
    c. Evaluation
    d. Diagnosis

14. Which statement best describes the evaluation phase of the nursing process?
    a. Subjective, objective, and psychosocial data are gathered in this phase.
    b. Nursing diagnoses are formulated during the evaluation phase.
    c. Evaluation happens across the continuum of the nursing process.
    d. This phase often begins with educating the patient on expected outcomes.

15. During the preoperative medication reconciliation process, the nurse discovers the patient's last dose of oral blood thinner medication was this morning. In reviewing the patient's chart, the nurse sees the patient received instruction to stop taking blood thinner medication seven days prior to the procedure. What is the most appropriate nursing action as a result of this information?
    a. Notify the surgeon and anesthesiologist that the patient received blood thinner up until this morning.
    b. Ask the patient why they continued to take the blood thinner after being instructed not to do so.
    c. Continue with the medication reconciliation process.
    d. Assess the patient's education level.

16. The medication reconciliation process includes which of the following components?
    a. Prescriber of medication
    b. Use of recreational drugs
    c. Only prescription medications
    d. Location of patient's preferred pharmacy

17. Ideally, the nurse utilizes which type of documentation, as it is considered best practice?
    a. Paper documentation
    b. Electronic medical record (EMR)
    c. Blended documentation
    d. Compartmentalized documentation

18. The goal of the nurse's preoperative patient assessment is to promote what?
    a. Best use of time and resources
    b. Cost-effectiveness
    c. Decreased turnover time
    d. Optimal patient outcomes and patient safety

19. The presence of body piercings and implanted foreign objects is noted in which phase of the preoperative plan of care?
    a. Planning
    b. Assessment
    c. Intervention
    d. Diagnosis

20. Which nursing intervention is appropriate during the immediate preoperative patient preparation process?
   a. Review of cardiac catheterization results
   b. Hair removal at surgical site
   c. Ordering pulmonary function tests
   d. Consideration of alternative treatment options

21. A patient's surgical procedure, date of birth, medication history, and previous medical procedures all constitute which of the following?
   a. The patient's electronic medical record
   b. Protected health information
   c. Records that can be provided to immediate family at any time
   d. Risk management tools

22. What is the purpose of the World Health Organization's (WHO's) Surgical Safety Checklist? Select the BEST answer.
   a. Increase patient safety throughout the perioperative spectrum.
   b. Reduce preoperative surgical risks.
   c. Reduce postoperative surgical risks.
   d. Replace perioperative checklists currently in place in surgical centers.

23. Which of the following details are necessary in order for checklists to be effective standardization tools?
   a. Checklists need to be aesthetically pleasing to the practitioner's eye, so that he or she is more likely to use it.
   b. Interdisciplinary team members must commit to using the checklist, and all members must use the checklist in the same context.
   c. Checklists need to be varied enough so that a diverse group of staff members has appropriate tasks (pertaining to their job role) to check off.
   d. A checklist must have a global presence in order to be considered a standardization tool.

24. Studies have shown that which of the following practices has the most positive impact on patients?
   a. Personalized comfort measures in their post-operation room, such as a favorite snack or book
   b. Internet and television access during their clinical stay
   c. An attentive communication style between their nurses and physicians
   d. Visible operation and safety checklists that staff members regularly check and notate

25. The registered nurse (RN) delegated the first step of the medication reconciliation process to the licensed practical nurse (LPN). Which action by the LPN signified understanding of this step?
   a. Ensured that all medication dosages are within therapeutic range by reviewing lab work
   b. Called the prescriber to clarify an order's dosage when handwriting is illegible
   c. Collected a complete medication history
   d. Documented each medication change and ensured it aligned with all other medication material

26. The nurse is completing a full body assessment. What should the nurse do after discovering illicit drugs in a small bag concealed in the patient's hair bun?
    a. Confiscate the drugs and report this finding to the police to let them decide how to proceed with the patient.
    b. Confiscate the drugs and page the nursing supervisor to elevate this concern.
    c. Send the illicit drugs home with the patient's spouse.
    d. Place the drugs in the patient's belonging bag that the security team monitors and releases back to the patient upon discharge.

27. During an abdominal physical assessment of a patient with gastrointestinal distress, which action should the nurse perform second?
    a. Percussion
    b. Auscultation
    c. Inspection
    d. Palpation

28. During a respiratory physical assessment of a patient with shortness of breath, which action should the nurse perform second?
    a. Inspection
    b. Percussion
    c. Palpation
    d. Auscultation

29. Which of the following is/are true regarding advance directives?
    a. They are an expression of the patient's preferences.
    b. They are based on a person's values and beliefs.
    c. They include identification of a surrogate.
    d. All of the above

30. While providing patient education, the nurse explains that the patient's medication dosage will need to be adjusted to find the most therapeutic level. What is this measured medication practice an example of?
    a. Medication compliance
    b. Medication reconciliation
    c. Medication titration
    d. Medication administration

31. Barbara suffered a fall in her living room. She landed on both hands with her arms outstretched, trying to brace for impact. Unfortunately, she felt immediate sharp pain in her right wrist, elbow, and shoulder. Her son drives her to the local emergency department for treatment. The local emergency department admits her, but decides to move her to a different facility in the same medical system due to overcapacity. They provide her with medication to manage the pain during transport. Upon arrival, the receiving clinical team should ask Barbara for which pieces of information before beginning treatment?
    a. Which facility she was sent from and what treatment she needs
    b. Her full name and full date of birth
    c. Her insurance information and weight
    d. Her date of birth and which medication she received at the first location

32. What is one critical benefit of implementing multi-modal pain therapies?
    a. Standardizing pain management across all patients
    b. Reducing total number of medications needed
    c. Reducing insurance costs
    d. Reducing adverse effects of opioids

33. Liam is about to undergo angioplasty and stent placement. Which of the following protocols may be helpful for Liam and his family to ensure Liam is the primary decision maker in unanticipated surgical situations?
    a. Advance directives
    b. Last will and testament
    c. Beneficiary designation
    d. Primary policyholder document

Individualized Plan of Care Development and Expected Outcomes

1. In an effort to promote perioperative patient safety, which government association imposes financial fees on organizations for negative patient outcomes such as stage III and IV pressure ulcers, surgical site infection (SSI), and retained foreign objects?
    a. Centers for Medicare and Medicaid Services (CMS)
    b. The Joint Commission (TJC)
    c. Institute of Medicine (IOM)
    d. World Health Organization (WHO)

2. Distractions such as background noise and conversations contribute to which type of human behavior errors?
    a. Skill based
    b. Knowledge based
    c. Situational
    d. Omission

3. Patient rights related to confidentiality and release of medical information are protected by what CMS product?
    a. Patient's Bill of Rights
    b. The WHO Surgical Safety Checklist
    c. The Health Insurance Portability and Accountability Act (HIPAA)
    d. TJC National Patient Safety Goals (NPSG)

4. In addition to patient rights, the patient has health care responsibilities. Which of the following is an example of patient responsibility related to medication management?
   a. The patient is responsible for disclosing use of prescription medications to the health care team, but not over-the-counter medications.
   b. The patient is responsible for using one pharmacy at a time, to decrease the chance of miscommunication of medication history between care providers.
   c. It is the responsibility of the patient to ensure prescribed medications are used by the patient only and are not given to family members for their use.
   d. The patient is responsible for knowing which medications combinations can potentially cause adverse reactions.

5. Regulatory bodies such as TJC and CMS clearly identify which need as one that must be fulfilled in order to promote optimal patient outcomes?
   a. Holistic care model
   b. Discharge planning
   c. Culturally based care
   d. Patient education

6. Being under obligation to provide safe patient care refers to what legal domain?
   a. Negligence
   b. Liability
   c. Standard of care
   d. Nurse Practice Act

7. How does each state board of nursing set the standards a nurse is expected to maintain in practice?
   a. Through its Nursing Practice Act
   b. By mandating a minimum number of continuing education units (CEUs) by nurses in all fifty states
   c. By defaulting to each institution's policies and procedures
   d. Individual states do not set these standards; federal guidelines govern these standards.

8. Public libraries and government offices are examples of which type of community resources?
   a. Local
   b. Demographical
   c. Institutional
   d. Geographical

9. In what situation would the Centers for Medicare and Medicaid Services (CMS) withhold reimbursement for patient care services provided by both a physician and health care institution?
   a. A patient is readmitted to the hospital with CHF exacerbation within thirty days of discharge for initial hospitalization for CHF management.
   b. A post-op coronary bypass graft (CABG) patient has an extended ventilator run due to chronic obstructive pulmonary disease (COPD) complications.
   c. The post-op abdominal aortic aneurysm patient is observed in the hospital one day longer than expected due to a history of renal failure.
   d. The patient with a history of coronary artery disease has post-op atrial fibrillation after colon resection surgery, warranting a cardiology consult.

10. Which is an example of how an electronic health record (EHR) improves patient outcomes?
   a. By reducing medical errors due to misinterpretation of handwriting
   b. By increasing the time a nurse spends researching the patient's disease process
   c. By decreasing the interdisciplinary team's access to patient information
   d. By discouraging the use of built-in systems in preventing treatment errors

11. What is recognized as the gold standard for preventing disease transmission?
   a. Antibiotic prophylaxis
   b. Decreasing surface contaminants in the patient's environment
   c. Screening patient visitors for communicable diseases
   d. Hand hygiene

12. Along with standard precautions, transmission-based precautions are used with patients with known or suspected infection with highly transmissible pathogens. What are the three categories of transmission-based precautions?
   a. Surface, droplet, and contact
   b. Contact, droplet, and airborne
   c. Surface, airborne, and contact
   d. Airborne, droplet, and surface

13. Which of the following is NOT a nursing intervention related to TJC's Surgical Care Improvement Project (SCIP) measures?
   a. Administering preoperative antibiotic prophylaxis as ordered
   b. Verifying blood products are available prior to surgical incision
   c. Applying antiembolism stockings
   d. Ensuring the patient has received beta-blocker medication as ordered within 24 hours of surgery

14. What task is reflective of the nurse considering the age-specific needs of a pediatric patient?
   a. Asking the chaplain to visit the elderly patient prior to entering the operating room
   b. Arranging an interpreter to be present during the adult's conversation with the surgeon
   c. Providing the toddler patient a stuffed animal
   d. Discussing postoperative pain management with the adolescent patient

15. What content is typically included in discharge instructions given to patients?

      I. Activities of daily living
      II. Nutrition plan
      III. When to call the doctor
      IV. New medications

   a. Choices I, III, and IV
   b. Choices II, III, and IV
   c. Choices I, II, and III
   d. All of the above

16. What should take place during a postoperative follow-up call by perioperative staff?
    a. Assess for any changes in health status, address patient and family concerns, validate medication regimen, and provide additional education.
    b. Conduct patient satisfaction surveys.
    c. Assess for changes in health status, but avoid excessive reinforcement education activities.
    d. Focus on positive postoperative outcomes instead of highlighting discrepancies in the patient's recovery.

17. Which of the following is an acronym used to remember and implement a comprehensive nursing handoff?
    a. MRSA
    b. STAR
    c. SBAR
    d. IPASS

18. A nine-year-old scheduled for a complex surgery is most likely to experience which of the following?
    a. Higher than normal amounts of parental anxiety, compared to other pediatric surgery patients
    b. The belief that they will wake up during the surgical process
    c. Separation anxiety from their parents
    d. Dissociation and lack of awareness of their surroundings

Intraoperative Activities

1. Which statement about infection control and hand hygiene is true?
    a. Hand hygiene is not necessary before donning sterile gloves in the perioperative environment.
    b. To be most effective, a two-minute hand wash should be performed after leaving the patient care area.
    c. The CDC reports healthcare providers clean their hands less than one half of the times they should.
    d. The spread of MDROs is not affected by hand washing.

2. Catheter-associated urinary tract infection (CAUTI) is a consideration for infection risk in the perioperative environment. Which patient DOES NOT meet the criteria for perioperative urinary catheter insertion?
    a. A fifty-seven-year-old male undergoing cardiac transplant
    b. An eighty-one-year-old female having a medication port insertion in order to begin chemotherapy
    c. A seventy-year-old female undergoing a bladder resection
    d. A thirty-nine-year-old undergoing femoral popliteal revascularization surgery

Use the following scenario to answer question 3.

John and Jennifer are preparing the operating room for a thoracotomy procedure. After donning surgical masks and ensuring traffic pattern is kept to a minimum, they begin to open sterile supplies into a sterile basin. Prior to opening each package, the integrity is checked, ensuring no holes or tears are present. After John opens a package of laparotomy sponges into the sterile basin, he inspects the package integrity and discovers a hole in the package.

3. What should John and Jennifer do after discovering the hole in the package?
   a. They should consider all the items in the sterile basin to be contaminated and discard them.
   b. They should consider only the contents that touched the laparotomy sponges in the basin to be contaminated and should carefully remove those contents with sterile forceps.
   c. Since the patient was not yet in the operating room, the sterile field is not yet established. They should proceed with opening sterile supplies into the basin.
   d. They should consider this surgery as a Class III (contaminated) case and alert infection control.

4. Which areas of the surgical gown are considered the sterile zones?
   a. The front (chest level to level of sterile field) and at the sleeves from two inches above the elbow to sleeve cuff
   b. The front (chest level to level of sterile field), at sleeves from two inches above elbow to sleeve cuff, and the back from two inches below neck to waistline
   c. The front (chest level to level of sterile field), at sleeves from shoulder to sleeve cuff, and the back from two inches below neck to waistline
   d. The front and back of gown, from neckline to waistline

5. Which of the following movements in and around the sterile field would contaminate the sterile field?
   a. The nonsterile perioperative nurse stands fifteen inches away from the sterile field to observe the procedure.
   b. The second circulating nurse exits the operating room through the door into the sterile hallway to obtain a surgical instrument from the instrument room.
   c. Midway through performing surgical skin prep, the nonsterile perioperative nurse walks between the patient and the sterile field to finish prepping the patient.
   d. The perioperative nurse utilizes a bag decanter to pour fluid into a sterile basin on the sterile field, being careful to not reach over the sterile field with her arm.

6. Which statement accurately describes an objective of skin prep antisepsis?
   a. Skin prep antisepsis is intended to sterilize the skin prior to surgery, decreasing the chance for SSI.
   b. Skin prep antisepsis inhibits rebound microorganism growth on the skin.
   c. By increasing the number of resident microorganisms on the skin, skin prep antisepsis prepares the body to defend itself against infectious bacteria.
   d. Removing visible soil and debris on the skin is the last step in skin prep antisepsis.

7. ChloraPrep is a commonly used chlorhexidine gluconate-based skin prep solution. For which patient is ChloraPrep solution contraindicated?

a. The forty-seven-year-old with a documented allergy to povidone iodine
b. The patient who has open venous stasis ulcers on the left lower extremity and is undergoing left leg revascularization
c. The patient with an intact left groin who is having a left groin hematoma evacuation
d. The open-heart surgery patient who has no open areas noted on the chest

8. Which statement is a reflection of the 1999 Institute of Medicine (IOM) report titled *To Err is Human: Building a Safer Health System*?

a. The IOM deleted the World Health Organization (WHO) surgical safety checklist as a result of the findings in the report.
b. The report found that patient safety is affected by one primary issue: inadequate hand hygiene compliance among healthcare professionals.
c. According to the report, addressing the objectives from the report requires action from the bedside caregiver but not hospital administrators.
d. As a result of the report, the IOM instituted six recommendations for improvement of patient safety: healthcare that is safe, effective, patient-centered, timely, efficient, and equitable.

9. How can the perioperative nurse manager implement safety guidelines to help minimize distraction and noise in the work environment?

a. Establish a no-distraction zone in medication preparation areas
b. Ask maintenance to decrease the set number of air exchanges in the operating room to decrease ventilation noise.
c. Eliminate traffic patterns in and out of the operating room once surgical incision is made.
d. Discourage the use of smoke evacuators, since the noise can distract the surgeon.

10. At what point in the perioperative nurse's employment should the healthcare institution's hazardous materials manual (HAZMAT) be introduced and reviewed?

a. At around six months after date of hire, to not overwhelm the nurse with too much educational material at once
b. At the beginning of employment
c. During annual mandatory education session only, because the information is not regularly updated
d. Only if the nurse is exposed to a hazardous chemical

11. The science of matching the physical requirements of a job to the physical abilities of the worker is known as what?

a. Physical dexterity
b. Body mechanics
c. Ergonomics
d. Foundational movement

12. In which nursing task would the perioperative nurse gain the MOST benefit from using safe patient mobilization (SPM) equipment?
  a. Applying a safety strap across the lower extremities to secure the patient to the operating room bed
  b. Rotating the operating room bed to the left per surgeon request
  c. Laterally transferring the patient from a stretcher to operating room bed
  d. Raising the head of the bed to provide orthopnea relief

13. To prevent hypothermia in perioperative patients, thermoregulation measures are implemented during procedures lasting longer than what duration?
  a. One hour
  b. Four hours
  c. Thirty minutes
  d. Two hours

14. Which of the following statements alerts the perioperative team to further investigate the patient's risk for developing malignant hyperthermia (MH)?
  a. The patient's preoperative lab testing shows an elevated serum potassium level.
  b. The patient reports a family history of complications with anesthesia.
  c. The patient's medical record indicates a history of postoperative nausea and vomiting.
  d. After reviewing the preoperative electrocardiogram (ECG), the cardiologist discovers the patient has a first-degree atrioventricular block.

15. Which members of the perioperative team are responsible for ensuring correct patient positioning?
  a. Perioperative nurse, anesthesiologist, and surgeon
  b. Anesthesiologist, perioperative nurse, and surgical technologist
  c. Perioperative nurse, surgeon, and surgical technologist
  d. Surgeon, anesthesiologist, and surgical technologist

16. Mr. Jones is scheduled for an abdominal aortic aneurysm repair. Which surgical position does the perioperative nurse anticipate for Mr. Jones?
  a. Lithotomy
  b. Left lateral
  c. Supine
  d. Kraske

17. When the patient's arms are positioned directly at the sides (tucked at the sides), the elbows are padded to protect against injury to which nerve?
  a. Sciatic nerve
  b. Vagus nerve
  c. Phrenic nerve
  d. Ulnar nerve

18. Which of the following patients is at HIGHEST risk for impaired postoperative wound healing, based on the given information?
    a. Mr. Jacob, a fifty-year-old with cardiomyopathy and Addison's disease
    b. Miss Kelly, a thirteen-year-old with Type I diabetes
    c. Mr. Davis, a seventy-six-year-old with gastroesophageal reflux disease (GERD) and hypothyroidism
    d. Mrs. Johnson, a twenty-nine-year-old with uncontrolled Type II diabetes and obesity

19. In which case is delayed primary closure indicated for achievement of wound healing?
    a. In the surgical case with an aseptically made wound with no tissue damage, because this is the preferred method for wound healing
    b. With collagen fibers present in the surgical wound
    c. In the case of compartment syndrome
    d. With cases involving the genitourinary tract

20. Dr. Johnson is completing the post procedure documentation for a patient who underwent a radical prostatectomy. No breaks in sterile technique occurred, and the wound is primarily closed. Which surgical wound class should be documented by Dr. Johnson?
    a. Class II (clean contaminated)
    b. Class IV (dirty/infected)
    c. Class III (contaminated)
    d. Class I (clean)

21. During a routine liver resection case, the perioperative nurse discovers one of the surgical instrument trays contains an indicator that does not pass sterility parameters. An abdominal retractor from this tray is being used on the patient. How should this case be identified, regarding surgical wound class?
    a. Class II (clean contaminated)
    b. Class III (contaminated)
    c. Class I (clean)
    d. Class IV (dirty/infected)

22. Which statement is MOST reflective of the importance of correctly identifying a surgical wound class?
    a. If the surgical wound class is not properly identified, an SSI may be improperly labeled as "hospital-acquired."
    b. Incorrect documentation of surgical wound class is likely to delay the patient's discharge from the hospital.
    c. Accurate identification of surgical wound class is important in predicting the patient's risk for postoperative hemorrhage.
    d. The Joint Commission (TJC) penalizes hospitals for performing Class IV surgeries.

23. Based on the American Society of Anesthesiologists (ASA) criteria for assessing patient health status prior to surgery, the patient with severe systemic disease that is not incapacitating, such as uncontrolled diabetes, is classified as belonging to which ASA category?
    a. ASA III
    b. ASA IV
    c. ASA V
    d. ASA VI

24. Spinal and epidural are types of which category of anesthesia?
    a. Monitored Anesthesia Care (MAC)
    b. Local
    c. Regional
    d. General

25. In order to be most effective, the patient's pain management plan is developed during which perioperative phase?
    a. Suboperative phase
    b. Intraoperative phase
    c. Postoperative phase
    d. Preoperative phase

26. Opioid analgesics work by binding to central nervous system receptors and tissues. Which medication is an example of an opioid analgesic?
    a. Ketorolac
    b. Succinylcholine
    c. Lidocaine
    d. Fentanyl

27. Which entry into the perioperative medication administration record contains all the necessary components of perioperative medication documentation?
    a. Lidocaine 0.25% administered subcutaneously at 1317 by J. Jones, MD.
    b. 2 mL of Lidocaine 0.25% administered subcutaneously at 1317 by J. Jones, MD.
    c. 2 mL of Lidocaine administered subcutaneously at 1317 by J. Jones, MD.
    d. 2 mL of Lidocaine 0.25% administered subcutaneously at 1317 by J. Jones, MD. Lidocaine expiration date 09/2020.

28. The perioperative charge nurse discovers a narcotic discrepancy in the medication dispensing system, Pyxis. According to Pyxis, seven vials of hydromorphone should be present, but there are only six. The charge nurse is unable to resolve the discrepancy with the last user who accessed the hydromorphone. What should the charge nurse's next step be in resolving the discrepancy?
    a. Report the discrepancy to pharmacy and/or hospital security.
    b. Adjust the Pyxis count and continue with other charge nurse duties, ignoring the discrepancy.
    c. Suggest unit-based education on the correct use of Pyxis.
    d. Retrieve hydromorphone from another Pyxis unit.

29. One use for surgical scissors is cutting suture material. Which of the following is another indicated use for surgical scissors?
    a. To clamp tissue together by using "teeth" that join together
    b. For visualization in minimally invasive procedures
    c. To provide traction away from the surgical area
    d. To dissect tissue for surgical exposure after skin incision is made

30. During a right leg revascularization procedure, the vascular surgeon needs to reduce blood flow at the surgical site during the proximal anastomosis, a critical point in the case. Which piece of surgical equipment would be the MOST helpful to the surgeon at this point?

a. Pneumatic tourniquet
b. X-ray detectable gauze
c. Surgical safety knife blade
d. Ventilator circuit

31. Which of the following is a type of surgical implant?

a. Nasogastric tube
b. Intravenous catheter
c. Mechanical heart valve
d: Indwelling urinary catheter

32. What statement is true regarding surgical implants?

a. If an infection develops after an item is surgically implanted, the implant is surgically removed, unless the surgeon deems it unsafe to remove the item.
b. Antibiotic prophylaxis is not indicated for the patient receiving a surgical implant, because the antibiotic can alter the patency of the implant.
c. Documentation of the surgical implant into the medical record includes the implant type, manufacturer brand and lot number, and the implant's cost to the patient.
d. Biological implant sources should not include human donors.

33. At worst, a retained surgical item can result in what patient event?

a. Increased hospital length of stay
b. Death
c. Increased cost of care
d. Minor infection

34. In accordance with best practice guidelines, at what points of care are surgical counts performed?

a. At the beginning of closure of body cavity or first tissue layer, during skin closure, and upon arrival to recovery unit
b. Prior to skin incision, at the beginning of closure of body cavity or first tissue layer, and during skin closure
c. Prior to skin incision, at the beginning of closure of body cavity or first tissue layer, during skin closure, and upon arrival at the recovery unit
d. Prior to skin incision and during skin closure

35. In which situation is it appropriate to omit the surgical count?

a. The patient with a ruptured abdominal aortic aneurysm has a blood pressure of 50/30 and is bleeding into the abdomen.
b. The patient with a left arm abscess is complaining of left arm pain and vital signs are stable.
c. The surgeon performing an open-heart procedure is in a hurry to get started, because he has two scheduled cases to complete.
d. The patient with lung cancer, whose DNR status is "no code," is having a chest tube inserted in the operating room.

36. Which of the following is an example of a surgical specimen?
  a. Electrosurgical unit (ESU) grounding pad
  b. Portion of left lower lobe of lung
  c. Metzenbaum scissors
  d. Operating room bed

37. A patient with hemoptysis presents to the operating room for a bronchoscopy. Upon visualization into the left mainstem bronchus, the surgeon sees an item that appears to be a thumb tack. The item is successfully removed. How should the specimen be labeled prior to sending it to pathology department for analysis?
  a. Thumb tack retrieved during bronchoscopy
  b. Hemoptysis-causing thumb tack
  c. Thumb tack
  d. Foreign body

38. Biohazardous materials are typically introduced into the perioperative environment in what forms?
  a. Autoclaves and carbon dioxide tanks
  b. Laser and ultraviolet radiation
  c. Cytotoxic and chemotherapy medications
  d. Patient body fluids and excreta

39. The types of perioperative hazards should FIRST be discussed at what point of the perioperative nurse's employment?
  a. At thirty days of employment
  b. After one year of employment
  c. After orientation is completed
  d. At the beginning of employment

40. How does surgical smoke, or a smoke plume, create a potential hazard for the perioperative team members?
  a. A smoke plume consists of anesthesia gases exhaled by the patient, causing potential sedation of surrounding perioperative team members.
  b. A smoke plume contains hazardous gases and biological material and can increase cancer risk for perioperative team members.
  c. A smoke plume causes thick smoke around the surgical site, causing decreased visibility of the surgical site.
  d. The presence of a smoke plume sets off the operating room's sprinkler system, contaminating the surgical field.

41. Which of the following BEST describes the Association of perioperative Registered Nurses (AORN) recommendation on the use of smoke evacuators to reduce the amount of surgical smoke?
   a. AORN recommends the use of smoke evacuators in all cases in which electrosurgical units (ESUs) and lasers are used.
   b. In cases lasting longer than four hours and in which an electrosurgical unit (ESU) or laser is used, AORN recommends the use of a smoke evacuator.
   c. AORN recommends using a smoke evacuator in cases involving use of an electrosurgical unit (ESU) or laser on a patient with a known communicable disease.
   d. AORN recommends using a smoke evacuator in cases using an electrosurgical unit (ESU) or laser on a patient with a cancer diagnosis.

42. Which of the following is an indication to reduce the operating room temperature below facility guidelines?
   a. The surgeon complains of being too warm.
   b. The patient is undergoing cardiopulmonary circulatory arrest.
   c. It is necessary to lower the patient's risk of developing SSI.
   d. The surgery is anticipated to last longer than one hour.

43. Humidity levels in the operating room are generally kept in which range?
   a. Between thirty and fifty percent
   b. Between twenty and sixty percent
   c. Between twenty and fifty percent
   d. Between thirty and sixty percent

44. How can the perioperative nurse safely and effectively contribute to reducing the level of noise in the operating room?
   a. Silence the telephone during critical points in the case.
   b. Use a muffling device on a noisy piece of equipment.
   c. Avoid unnecessary conversations.
   d. Stop room traffic during critical periods of the case.

45. For patients receiving anticoagulation therapy, which two laboratory values may be tested to determine the need for anticoagulation reversal agents?
   a. Protime/international normalized ratio (PT/INR) and partial thromboplastin time (PTT)
   b. Protime/international normalized ratio (PT/INR) and hemoglobin
   c. Partial thromboplastin time (PTT) and hematocrit
   d. Protime/international normalized ratio (PT/INR) and blood urea nitrogen (BUN)

46. Which of the following is often used in cases in which a high amount of blood loss is anticipated?
   a. Cryoprecipitate transfusion
   b. ABO uncrossmatched blood
   c. Intraoperative cell salvage
   d. Platelet therapy

47. In areas where surgical equipment is in use, The Joint Commission (TJC) and The Centers for Medicare and Medicaid Services (CMS) require the presence of what document related to equipment use?

a. World Health Organization (WHO) equipment safety checklist
b. The United States Food and Drug Administration (FDA) equipment manual
c. Manufacturer's instructions for use (IFU)
d. Surgical Care Improvement Project (SCIP) equipment log

48. Which governing body is responsible for testing medical equipment and approving it for safe patient use?

a. The United States Food and Drug Administration (FDA)
b. The Centers for Medicare and Medicaid Services (CMS)
c. The Joint Commission (TJC)
d. The Occupational Safety and Health Administration (OSHA)

49. If the IFU for a piece of surgical equipment indicates the equipment poses a potential fire hazard, what recommendation for protecting the patient and equipment users can the perioperative nurse expect to find in the IFU?

a. The type of intravenous fluids to administer during the case
b. The type of warming blanket to use on the patient
c. The amount of x-ray detectable gauze to have on the surgical field
d. The type of fire extinguisher that should be available

50. Which observation should prompt the circulator to speak up?

a. A surgery resident making the initial incision for the procedure under supervision
b. An RNFA performing the surgical time-out
c. The primary surgeon's fellow closing the incision
d. An x-ray technician entering the OR

51. Which of the following statements is true about recycling in the OR?

a. Should never take place due to the risk of infection
b. May be possible for certain types of materials
c. Depends on the surgeon's preference
d. Applies to all types of materials used

52. What should product selection in the OR be based on?

a. Cost alone
b. Surgeon's preference alone
c. Product's efficacy alone
d. A combination of cost, effectiveness, and surgeon preferences

53. When should family members be allowed in the OR?

a. Under no circumstances
b. In some cases
c. For all pediatric procedures
d. Whenever they request

54. Which of the following statements is true?
    a. Terminal cleaning should ideally be completed at the end of the day.
    b. Terminal cleaning must be completed between every case.
    c. Terminal cleaning is only required after a patient on isolation precautions has been in the room.
    d. Terminal cleaning should ideally be completed at the beginning of every day of scheduled cases.

55. While being stored in the OR, when should a heart valve tissue implant's temperature indicator be checked for compliance?
    a. Daily
    b. At the time of implant only
    c. Both on receipt of the tissue and at the time of implant
    d. When the facility receives the tissue

56. When are N-95 masks required when caring for a patient?
    a. Patient has been diagnosed with MRSA.
    b. Patient has been diagnosed with tuberculosis.
    c. Patient has been diagnosed with VRE.
    d. Patient has been diagnosed with *C. difficile.*

57. The circulator is preparing for a case that requires use of a microscope at the midpoint of the procedure. When should the circulator check on the microscope's availability?
    a. At the midpoint of the procedure when the microscope is needed
    b. At the time of incision
    c. At the time of induction
    d. Before the patient enters the OR

58. When should product evaluation and selection take place?
    a. Annually with the interdisciplinary team
    b. Annually with only surgeons
    c. Ad hoc with the interdisciplinary team
    d. Ad hoc with only surgeons

59. When is vendor supervision required?
    a. It is always required
    b. It is only required if the vendor is new
    c. It is only required if the surgeon requests
    d. It is never required

60. Which statement is true about environmental sustainability practices?
    a. Due to possible contamination, it is not possible to reprocess or recycle any materials or equipment.
    b. Countable items that are eligible for reprocessing can be removed from the room during the case.
    c. Some equipment and materials may be reprocessed or recycled depending on the facility's policies.
    d. Visibly soiled items from the case can be reprocessed or recycled.

61. What personal protective equipment (PPE) should be changed in between cases?
    a. Hair covering
    b. Any PPE that is visibly soiled
    c. Scrubs
    d. Shoe covers

62. In the event of a spill, what should the circulator do?
    a. Refer to the OSHA manual if unsure how to clean the spill.
    b. Immediately request assistance from the turnover cleaning staff.
    c. Not clean the spill until the case is completed.
    d. Only clean if the spill is in proximity to the sterile field.

63. Which of the following statements is true about preventive maintenance of equipment?
    a. It is the responsibility of the biomedical engineering department and has no impact on the nursing staff.
    b. It is a team effort, and the circulator should communicate with the appropriate parties to ensure equipment is available for upcoming cases.
    c. It does not require advance planning.
    d. It should not take place; equipment should only be serviced if it is inoperable so that it is always available for procedures.

64. An implant is used during a case that has paperwork for the manufacturer. Which of the following is true for this paperwork?
    a. It does not need to be completed if the circulator is documenting the implant information in the patient's medical record.
    b. It should be completed only if the circulator has enough time during the case.
    c. It should be completed and kept in the patient's medical record.
    d. It should be completed and returned to the manufacturer.

65. Which of the following statements is true about the fluid used to reconstitute a tissue?
    a. It should be included in the implant documentation.
    b. It should be lactated Ringer's solution.
    c. It does not need to be sterile.
    d. It can be any fluid already on the sterile field.

66. Which of the following would NOT indicate possible contamination of an instrument tray?
    a. Moisture in the bottom of the outer pan of an autoclaved instrument tray
    b. A hole in the paper filter of the tray top
    c. A tear in the count sheet paper
    d. An incomplete sterile indicator

67. When should equipment for the second case of the day ideally be confirmed?
    a. Prior to the day of surgery
    b. The morning of surgery
    c. After the incision has been made on the first case
    d. After the first case has been completed

68. When should the nursing team monitor for changes to regulatory guidelines and recommendations?
    a. Annually
    b. Quarterly
    c. Only when it contradicts the facility's policies and procedures
    d. Constantly

69. Which of the following psychosocial occupational hazards are nurses at high risk of experiencing in the operating room?
    a. Lumbar strains
    b. Compassion fatigue
    c. Codependency
    d. Needle sticks

70. Nurses can help patients have the best surgical outcomes by recommending that the patient abstains from which of the following at least forty-eight hours prior to a procedure?
    a. Exercise
    b. Naps
    c. Alcohol
    d. Group activities

71. Bram goes to a routine annual physical and learns that he has stage II colon cancer. While his prognosis is favorable, he will need to undergo several rounds of chemotherapy and radiation. He shares this news with his employer, who helps Bram complete leave of absence paperwork for a two-week period followed by approval for an indefinite work-from-home period. A week later, Bram receives a letter from his employer-sponsored health insurance company saying that due to his recent diagnosis, his plan is changing to a more comprehensive plan with more expansive coverage but a higher annual deductible. Of which law is the insurance company in violation?
    a. Patient Protection and Affordable Care Act
    b. Consolidated Omnibus Budget Reconciliation Act
    c. Health Insurance Portability and Accountability Act
    d. Americans with Disabilities Act

72. Healthcare providers that specialize in surgery have over twice the rate of which health issue, compared to the general population?
    a. Burnout
    b. Heart disease
    c. Overweight or obesity
    d. Musculoskeletal injuries

73. Surgical skin prep significantly reduces the chances of the patient experiencing which of the following?
    a. Anxiety
    b. Unanticipated tearing
    c. Infection
    d. Adverse anesthetic outcomes

74. Joe is a perioperative nurse readying a sterile field in an operating room. He is preparing to add equipment to the field. He has a sealed sponge forceps that needs to be included in the sterile field for the attending surgeon. How should Joe place the forceps into the sterile field?

a. Place the sealed package onto the field, and allow the surgeon to open it at the time of need.
b. Face the package away and peel the seal from the farthest corner; drop the forceps into the sterile field at a gentle angle.
c. Remove the forceps and place the end into a sterile bag; set the bagged portion into the sterile field so that the handle of the forceps can be grabbed easily.
d. Open the package, wipe down the forceps with an antiseptic wipe, and place in the center of the sterile field.

75. Which of the following is an example of a Class III wound?

a. A scratch on the cornea from a sterile contact lens
b. A surgical site in the rectum
c. A puncture in the foot after stepping on a nail
d. An endoscopic incision for esophageal surgery

Communication and Documentation

1. Perioperative interviews may take place in which of the following settings?

I. Surgeon's office
II. Outpatient surgical center
III. Operating room
IV. Telephonically

a. Choices I, II, and IV
b. Choices II and III
c. Choices I, II, and III
d. All of the above

2. Patient S. will undergo a laparoscopic procedure that is going to require conscious sedation. During the perioperative interview, Patient S. reveals to the nurse that he currently does not have any transportation to get home following his procedure. What actions should the perioperative nurse take?

a. Document the lack of transportation as being a risk postoperatively and notify the surgeon the day of the procedure.
b. There is no need to document the lack of transportation, but the nurse will need to notify the physician.
c. Document that the patient will not have transportation following the procedure, notify the physician, and discuss possible transportation alternatives with the patient.
d. Encourage the patient to find someone who can pick him up following the procedure and move on to the next question.

3. Clinical information technology is associated with which of the following?

a. Clinical tasks
b. Admissions
c. Pharmacy
d. Laboratory

4. Which of the following is an advantage associated with information technology in the perioperative setting?
    a. Increase in the use of clinical pathways
    b. Reduction in the accessibility to quality health care
    c. Cost savings
    d. Concise paper charting

5. Nurse Jones is the circulating nurse during a myomectomy procedure in which six fibroids are removed from a patient's uterus. One of the fibroids is 8 cm in diameter. She takes a picture of the fibroid and posts it to her social media page. What are the possible ramifications for Nurse Jones' actions?
    a. There are no ramifications for Nurse Jones as long as she does not mention the patient's name.
    b. The nurse may receive a suspension or termination notice, and the facility may also receive a significant fine.
    c. The nurse may receive a fine, but the facility will not be held accountable for the actions of one person.
    d. Nurse Jones will not be punished, but the facility will lose its accreditation.

6. Which of the following is a method that may be utilized to track processes and procedures while also serving as a communication tool among multiple disciplines?
    a. Perioperative checklist
    b. Policies and procedures
    c. Clinical pathway
    d. Perioperative workflow

7. A medical teaching hospital experienced three errors over four months. All errors were directly caused by first-year residents. The teaching hospital chooses to report these errors, though they aren't required to do so. Patient information is noted but kept confidential. Under which legal act do these actions fall?
    a. HIPAA
    b. FAFSA
    c. PSQIA
    d. ADA

8. In a clinical setting, when are patients most likely to experience inadequate care or adverse effects to their overall health status?
    a. During or after a hand-off or transition between staff members
    b. Upon discharge
    c. When completing reimbursement paperwork
    d. When trying to complete basic functions like eating or using the restroom

9. Jonah is a support nurse who is managing the care of a post-operative cardiac patient. On the morning that the patient is to be discharged, Jonah notices that the patient suddenly has an erratic heart rhythm and a slight increase in blood pressure. The patient says to Jonah, "I feel great! I can't wait to get home; you can see that I'm excited about it!" However, Jonah pages a nurse practitioner and the attending physician. He tells them that he's worried about the change in the patient's cardiac functioning and doesn't think the patient should be discharged. What technique is Jonah utilizing to communicate his worries?

a. I PASS the BATON
b. SBAR
c. CUS
d. TeamSTEPPS

10. What information is usually discussed during a pre-operative interview?

a. What the patient is most nervous about and the lifestyle behaviors that contributed to the operation
b. The patient's demographic information, medical history, review of the procedure, pre-operation requirements, discharge and post-operative requirements, and any last-minute questions the patient might have
c. Detailed discussions of case studies relating to the procedure and the different outcomes that can result in order to prepare the patient for all outcomes
d. The patient's financial status, the type of insurance coverage they carry, the patient's financial responsibility at check-in and discharge, and where to get financial assistance if needed

11. Which of these situations often cause a barrier to effective communication between nurses?

a. Physical disability
b. A busy work setting and the consequent need to multitask
c. Above-average rate of colleague absences, as compared to other industries
d. None of the above

12. Amy is a nurse practitioner that has begun her shift. Using her designated log-in, she signs into a mobile clinical workstation and reviews how many patients are scheduled for appointments with her during this shift. She notices that her first patient has already been checked in by the front-desk staff, so she logs out of the workstation and greets her patient. Once roomed, Amy logs back into the room's clinical workstation and pulls up the patient's medical history and chief complaint to review with him. The patient mentions he has a new allergy to NSAIDs, which Amy documents in his electronic medical record. Later, the patient goes to the clinic's pharmacy to pick up a prescription that Amy ordered. The pharmacist is able to note the patient's updated allergy information and double-checks that the patient's prescription won't cause any issues. He also provides the patient with a patient portal log-in so that the patient can order a refill when he's out of his current medication. What primary tool is the medical organization effectively utilizing to streamline processes, improve documentation, and enhance accessibility to care?

a. Healthcare information technology
b. Paper charting documentation
c. A nearby pharmacy
d. A customer-service oriented pharmacist

13. After a long day in trauma surgery cases, nurses Lana and Mike eat a quick dinner together and head to their respective homes. Lana logs into her social media account and posts a message that she had a tiring day at work due to a complicated gunshot wound case. Mike replies to her post, "I'm so glad that our patient made it! He was just a kid, and I was really worried. That wound really messed up the cool bird tattoo on his right leg, though!" Both messages can be seen by any of Lana and Mike's common friends who also use this social media platform. This exchange is a violation of which of the following?
   a. All of JHCO best practices
   b. Digital media copyright laws
   c. HIPAA
   d. PSQIA

14. Which of the following is NOT a benefit of perioperative education?
   a. It may reduce patient anxiety regarding the procedure.
   b. It can foster a positive, trusting relationship between the patient and the nurse.
   c. It may reduce the overall length of the patient's stay.
   d. It ensures that the patient won't have an adverse relapse after the procedure.

15. What non-clinical areas may nurses find themselves assisting with in order to support the overall efficiency of organizational processes?
   a. Project management, business analyses, and/or software development
   b. Cleaning, sanitizing, and/or sweeping surfaces
   c. Telemedicine, telenursing, and/or virtual healthcare delivery
   d. Curriculum development and/or teaching nursing students

16. Which of the following are common distractions that can adversely impact the hand-off process?
   a. Low patient census
   b. Slow-pace environment
   c. Surgeon engagement
   d. High patient census and rapid turnovers

17. Which of the following is a characteristic of a good hand-off?
   a. One-way communication
   b. Repetitive and brief
   c. Specific
   d. Involves multiple care providers

18. Which of the following is a concern that a nurse would escalate to the surgeon?
   a. Normal laboratory values
   b. Patient not understanding postoperative care needs
   c. Pain management plan and schedule
   d. Family care plan for patient after discharge

19. How can perioperative nursing staff best help children prepare for an upcoming procedure?
   a. Avoid providing too much detail about the procedure or what to expect to reduce the risk of anxiety.
   b. Stay away from empathetic behaviors with the child, as this can make the child more fearful of the surgery or outcome.
   c. Introduce the child to terminology and equipment that they might encounter within the perioperative setting such as IVs, oxygen masks, and monitors.
   d. Limit exposure to the perioperative setting to the day of surgery.

20. What are the advantages of providing perioperative patient education before surgery?
      I. Reduction in the length of stay
      II. Fewer pain medication interventions
      III. Increase in patient or patient-family satisfaction
      IV. Increase in the retention of information provided

   a. Choices I, III, and IV
   b. Choices II and III
   c. Choices I, II, and III
   d. All of the above

21. What is the potential risk of providing patient education the same day of a procedure?
   a. Gaps in patient understanding
   b. Increased patient satisfaction
   c. Repetitive information from multiple sources
   d. Delays in care

22. A surgery center is borrowing an instrument from a neighboring hospital. The instrument is sealed in a sterile package upon arrival. What should be done before using the instrument?
   a. The instrument is sterile and can be used immediately.
   b. Contact the neighboring hospital to verify sterility.
   c. Resterilize the instrument before use.
   d. Log the instrument for tracking and deliver it to the OR nurse.

23. What is one benefit of electronic health records?
   a. They can be accessed across multiple medical facilities.
   b. They can be accessed internationally, as many countries have adopted the same system.
   c. They require minimal training to adopt.
   d. They can be easily accessed in areas with limited internet service, such as rural areas.

24. Which of the following is generally **not** included in patient discharge care?
   a. Information to prevent infection
   b. A plan for patient transportation to their home
   c. Prescription information
   d. Prior authorization paperwork

25. A natural disaster, internet outage, software glitch, and mass casualty event can all result in which of the following?
    a. Improved patient access
    b. Triage
    c. Downtime
    d. An increase in tetanus vaccinations

Infection Prevention and Control

1. What solutions should be used to keep instruments free of bioburdens?
    a. Saline
    b. Sterile water
    c. Tap water
    d. Lactated Ringer's solution

2. How long should sterilization monitoring records remain on file (at a minimum)?
    a. One year
    b. Two years
    d. Three years
    d. Four years

3. Which class of disinfectants require Food and Drug Administration (FDA) approval?
    a. Low-level
    b. Intermediate-level
    c. High-level
    d. Any disinfectant used in a medical setting requires FDA approval.

4. According to the Spaulding Classification System, what type of instruments is classified as critical?
    a. Instruments that enter sterile tissue or anywhere in the vascular system
    b. Instruments that enter only mucous membranes
    c. Instruments that make contact with the skin
    d. Instruments that make contact with high-level disinfectants

5. What's the probability that a potentially dangerous microorganism will survive on a properly sterilized medical instrument?
    a. 1 in 1,000
    b. 1 in 10,000
    c. 1 in 100,000
    d. 1 in 1,000,000

6. According to the Spaulding Classification System, blood pressure cuffs are an example of what type of instrument?
    a. A critical item
    b. A non-critical item
    c. A reliable item
    d. A monitoring item

7. Which of the following disinfecting agents is highly effective in small amounts, one of the strongest disinfectants used in healthcare institutions, relatively safe for workers, and powerful in low temperatures?
   a. Sodium peroxide
   b. Sodium Hypochlorite
   c. Formaldehyde
   d. Hydrogen peroxide

8. What is one of the oldest, cheapest, and chemical-free sterilization methods still used in healthcare settings?
   a. Wiping with microfiber towels
   b. Steam sterilization
   c. Infrared sterilization
   d. Freeze-motivated sterilization

9. Micah is assisting with the surgery of a patient who has a shoulder injury. A medical device is being implanted in the patient's shoulder. Micah retrieves the sterile package in which the medical device is held. As Micah turns to hand it to the surgeon, he trips on his surgical bootie and the package falls on the floor but does not open. Micah quickly changes his gloves, picks up the package, and the surgery continues. What is the main cause for concern in this case?
   a. The package fell on the floor, which means it may no longer be considered sterile and should not be used in the surgery.
   b. A patient with a shoulder injury should never receive an implanted device.
   c. Micah shouldn't have changed his gloves at any time during the case.
   d. Another team member should have retrieved the package and Micah should have been excused to ensure there was no serious reason behind his fall.

10. Which of the following is NOT a common standard precaution used to mitigate cross-contamination and/or mixing of bodily fluids?
   a. Washing hands thoroughly, properly, and regularly
   b. Disposing of syringes and other sharp objects in designated, secure storage sites
   c. Requiring that all clinical staff keep personal hand sanitizer bottles on their person while on a shift
   d. Wearing gloves and changing gloves between patients

11. Aria is a nurse who primarily works with breast cancer patients. She is working with a new patient who will be undergoing chemotherapy, and Aria is waiting for physician's orders as to how the patient's treatment plan will proceed. The physician arrives and seems distressed. She quickly reviews the new patient's file and tells Aria that the first chemotherapy treatment can take place the following day. Then the physician hurries off. What would be the best course of action for Aria in order to ensure her new patient begins treatment as soon as possible?
   a. Make sure that she receives written and signed orders from the physician on a chemotherapy order form.
   b. Follow up with the physician to ask if anything is wrong in the physician's personal life.
   c. Check with the patient if the patient is available for an appointment the next day, and if the patient has reliable transportation to and from the facility.
   d. Begin treatment on the patient now, as the patient is already at the center and Aria is a seasoned nurse who knows how to proceed with the patient's treatment.

12. If a loaned instrument is brought into a facility from an outside source, what's the first step it will undergo upon arrival?

a. It will be physically checked by the physician who will be using it.
b. It will be kept in a temperature-controlled holding room for seven days.
c. It will be inspected by a representative from its manufacturing company.
d. It will be sterilized and tagged as a loaned instrument.

13. Which of the following characteristics are preferable for an area that serves as a storage location for sterile equipment?

a. An open shelving area that can be easily accessed when the instrument is needed
b. A humid, empty room that can be locked
c. A dry, temperature-controlled room that has limited staff access
d. Bright environments with a lot of natural sunlight, to provide ease of instrument selection for staff members

14. Which of the following is the best way to prevent the spread of infection?

a. Keeping the mouth covered when coughing or sneezing
b. Disinfecting shared patient equipment
c. Practicing proper hand hygiene
d. Avoiding contact with infectious patients

15. A patient has just had abdominal surgery with a large incision site. The nurse knows that which of the following is *not* a sign that the wound has become infected?

a. Redness
b. Coolness
c. Heat
d. Swelling

16. When reviewing their knowledge of the stages of infections, the nurse knows that which period precedes the first symptoms of the infection?

a. Prodromal period
b. Colonization of organism
c. Incubation period
d. Convalescent period

17. When reducing the risk of infection transmission, which personal protective equipment (PPE) should the nurse don first?

a. Gloves
b. Mask
c. Gown
d. Goggles

18. Which approach to doffing personal protective equipment (PPE) supports infection control?

a. Removing PPE at the nursing station
b. Removing PPE at the bedside immediately following use
c. Removing PPE in the patient's bathroom
d. Removing PPE at the patient's doorway

19. An aide is caring for a patient with a known respiratory infection. The patient is on droplet precautions. What is the minimum PPE required when caring for this patient?
    a. Gloves, gown, N-95 respirator
    b. Gown, eyewear, gloves, and a disposable mask
    c. Gloves and a disposable mask
    d. Disposable mask, sterile gloves, and eyewear

20. Perioperative inoculation of bacteria into the joint describes which of the following?
    a. A post-op infection
    b. A prosthetic joint infection
    c. Infectious arthritis
    d. All of the above

21. Which infection control precautions should the medical-surgical nurse implement to reduce the risk of transmission for a patient diagnosed with active tuberculosis?
    a. Standard
    b. Contact
    c. Droplet
    d. Airborne

22. How often should terminal cleaning of the operating room occur?
    a. Every 24 hours
    b. After every surgical procedure
    c. Before a high-risk surgery
    d. Only when a patient is at risk for infection

23. Which of the following instruments requires postoperative sterilization to prevent surgical site infections?
    a. Rectal scope
    b. Scalpel
    c. Axillary thermometer
    d. Laryngoscope blade

24. A charge nurse is performing an environmental check in the surgical equipment storage room. The nurse accidentally tears the package of single-use surgical forceps. Which action does the nurse perform next?
    a. Clean the forceps with a high-level disinfectant
    b. Prepare the forceps for sterilization
    c. Discard the forceps
    d. Place the forceps in a new wrapper

25. A supervisory nurse has completed daily monitoring of sterilization procedures. Which indicator will NOT be part of the documentation?
    a. Mechanical
    b. Clinical
    c. Biological
    d. Chemical

26. A specimen containing a genital swab obtained during surgery will be transported to the laboratory in a bag of which color?
    a. Green
    b. Blue
    c. Red
    d. Black

27. A nurse is monitoring a surgical technologist who is disposing of biohazard waste into a bag after a surgical procedure. The nurse will intervene if they observe the surgical tech discard which item into the bag?
    a. Glove
    b. Gown
    c. Syringe
    d. Scalpel

28. A surgeon orders post hardware placement x-rays on a patient. The nurse must ensure that surgical team members are wearing which personal protective equipment?
    a. Goggles
    b. N-95 mask
    c. Lead apron
    d. Sterile gloves

29. Which chemical monitoring test is used to assess the functionality of a steam sterilizer's vacuum system?
    a. Bowie-Dick
    b. Rapid-readout ETO
    c. 16-Towel
    d. Spore

30. A nurse is inspecting the surgical storage room. Which observation compromises the sterility of surgical instruments and supplies?
    a. Packages are stored 20 inches from the ceiling.
    b. Packages are stacked on top of each other.
    c. The temperature in the room is 70 °F (21.1 °C).
    d. The humidity in the room is 50%.

31. A surgeon has requested an instrument that is unavailable in the operating room. An outside facility will be loaning the instrument. Which process ensures that the instrument is returned to the outside facility postoperatively?
    a. Documenting a note in the operative record
    b. Informing the supervisory nurse of the loaned instrument
    c. Assigning an OR staff member to secure the instrument
    d. Tagging the instrument when it arrives at the facility

32. A nurse notes a surgical technologist wearing a hair cover and surgical scrubs while at the scrub station. Which other surgical attire will the nurse instruct the surgical tech to apply?
   a. Gown
   b. Sterile gloves
   c. Mask
   d. Lead apron

33. A vascular surgeon is working an emergency department shift and supporting the care of trauma patients. Her day is booked full of scheduled cases, and the nursing staff are working diligently to keep incoming emergency cases stabilized until the surgeon is able to see them. Which of the following is the surgery team required to complete in between these cases?
   a. Financial counseling with the patient or family member
   b. Room turnover
   c. Taking 30-minute lunch breaks on staggered shifts
   d. Ensuring that non-clinical staff are managing software updates

34. Michael is a surgical nurse preparing for his team's first case of the day. He goes to the patient's hospital room and asks both the patient and the patient's family members how they are doing and if they have any questions or concerns about the procedure or the patient's stay. After speaking with them, Michael heads to the operating room. Prior to entering, he scrubs his hands following operating hand hygiene protocol; then, he dons a surgical mask, hair cover, and beard cover. The patient is anesthetized and wheeled into the room, where Michael documents the patient's condition upon arrival and confirms that all medical equipment is out and prepared for the procedure. During the procedure, an additional scalpel is needed. Michael retrieves the scalpel, and using sterile technique, presents the additional scalpel to the surgeon. Once the procedure is finished, Michael tallies all of the equipment used alongside the open packages. Ensuring that all equipment is present, he documents a form and lets the surgery team know that all equipment has been accounted for. As the patient is wheeled out of the operating room, Michael prepares for room turnover, discards his used protective gear, washes his hands, and heads out to meet with the patient's family. What official title does Michael likely hold?
   a. Scrub nurse
   b. Circulating nurse
   c. Nurse anesthetist
   d. Sterile compounding technician

35. Shoe covers are required in which zones of a medical facility?
   a. Restricted zones only
   b. Restricted and semi-restricted zones
   c. Unrestricted zones
   d. Semi-restricted zones only

36. During which of the following situations would hand hygiene using an alcohol-based hand sanitizer be appropriate?
   a. Upon noticing a small paper cut on one's hand
   b. After using the restroom
   c. After touching something that may contain a fungal spore
   d. After removing one's personal protective gloves

Emergency Situations

1. Jaw clenching, tachycardia, flushed skin, and muscle rigidity during a surgical procedure are all indicative of which emergency?
   a. Fainting
   b. Lung puncture
   c. Malignant hyperthermia
   d. Extreme depressive episode

2. What is the immediate course of action when a patient shows symptoms of malignant hyperthermia during surgery?
   a. Pour ice cold water over the patient and place cool cloths on the patient's forehead.
   b. Administer dantrolene at a dose of 2.5 mg/kg.
   c. Administer electrolytes at a solution of 3 mg/kg.
   d. Halt surgery and prepare to defibrillate the patient.

3. Penicillin, latex, propofol, and iodine contrast dye are common triggers of which emergency situation that can present in the operating room?
   a. Malignant hypothermia
   b. Stroke
   c. Seizures
   d. Anaphylaxis

4. Which condition is a common secondary event that occurs as a direct result of another emergency condition in a patient?
   a. Excessive sleepiness
   b. Cardiac arrest
   c. Edema
   d. Permanent paralysis

5. Patient X is scheduled for surgery and has a history of anesthesia complications during two previous surgeries. The medical team feels Patient X is at a high risk of developing malignant hyperthermia during the procedure. How should the team prepare?
   a. Keep a minimum of 36 units of dantrolene and enough sterile water available during the entirety of the procedure.
   b. Cancel the patient's operation and recommend that the patient schedules the operation at a Level 3 Trauma Center instead.
   c. Complete the surgery in parts over a course of multiple days.
   d. Inform the patient that the overall prognosis looks grim.

6. Which of the following tasks is NOT the responsibility of the circulator (circulating nurse)?
   a. Delegating specific tasks to team members
   b. Communicating to all team members in the event of a natural disaster or environmental threat, and coordinating safety and evacuations efforts for the team and the patient
   c. Ensuring the patient's insurance paperwork is accurate and up to date
   d. Ensuring the "crash cart" is stocked and ready

7. What three primary components cause a surgical fire?
   a. An oxidizer, an ignition source, and a fuel source
   b. Poor medical staff awareness, poor lighting, and a lack of a fire extinguisher
   c. Sodium peroxide, sodium dioxide, hydrogen peroxide
   d. Cigarettes, lighters, gasoline

8. What indicators do most medical facilities use to code emergency situations?
   a. Colors
   b. Numbers
   c. Locations
   d. Shapes

9. Which of the following may be used to treat anaphylactic patients?
   a. Augmentin
   b. Epinephrine
   c. Amoxicillin
   d. Electroshock therapy

10. A hospital located on the Florida panhandle reviews evacuation protocol at the beginning and middle of every hurricane season. What document does this hospital likely review with its staff members?
   a. Hospital flood insurance policies
   b. A published disaster plan
   c. Fire drill safety locations
   d. How to receive free ride-sharing credits to use in the event of a hurricane

11. What tool can be utilized to reduce or eliminate toxic fumes in the operating room?
   a. A fire extinguisher
   b. An open-valve oxygen tank
   c. A smoke evacuator
   d. A carbon monoxide detector

12. Crash carts are most commonly needed to treat which types of patients?
   a. Pregnant patients
   b. Patients experiencing cardiac arrest
   c. Elderly patients
   d. Pediatric patients

13. What is the primary role of a scrub technician?
   a. To fully prepare an operating room for a procedure, including, but not limited to, preparing all equipment and ensuring the cleanliness and safety of the room
   b. To aid all team personnel in scrubbing in and completing a checklist to ensure all sanitary measures have been performed by each team member
   c. To float and offer support as needed to nursing staff during the surgical procedure
   d. To administer anesthesia

14. Which of these commonly used surgical tools can start an operating room fire?
   a. A scalpel
   b. A heating pad
   c. An electrocautery pencil
   d. A smoke evacuator

15. A surgical team based in Los Angeles is about to begin a procedure when a sudden, fairly large earthquake hits. The team is about to perform a life-sustaining operation on a cardiac patient. The patient is already under general anesthesia. What should the team do?
   a. Keep working, as the surgery is life-sustaining
   b. As they haven't begun the procedure, the team should quickly evacuate, bringing all the items necessary to sustain the patient with them.
   c. Seek cover for themselves and the patient and begin the procedure when the earthquake subsides; if another tremor occurs, they should cover the surgical wound and move the patient.
   d. Each team member should protect themselves and run to safety.

16. What is an environmental safety risk during laparoscopic surgeries?
   a. The laparoscope can get stuck in the patient's dermal layer.
   b. The laparoscope is likely to short circuit the room unless it's initially connected to a small generator.
   c. The laparoscope's light cord can potentially cause a fire, especially if it comes in contact with surgical drapes or alcohol-based equipment.
   d. Laparoscopes used to be risky when they were initially introduced but now use advanced technologically to be virtually risk-free.

17. Which of these allergies can be hereditary and cause complications during surgical procedures?
   a. Perfume-related allergies
   b. Animal dander allergies
   c. Copper and nickel allergies
   d. Latex allergies

18. The patient with primary hypertension is being treated with medications to reduce blood volume and lower systemic vascular resistance. Which of the following medication combinations should the nurse anticipate for the patient?
   a. A diuretic and a calcium channel blocker (CCB)
   b. A diuretic and an angiotensin-converting enzyme (ACE) inhibitor
   c. An angiotensin II receptor blocker (ARB) and morphine
   d. A diuretic and a beta-blocker

19. Which of the following is a contraindication for thrombolytic therapy?
   a. Current anticoagulant therapy
   b. Over age 75
   c. Severe hepatic disease
   d. INR of 3.5

20. A patient involved in a motor vehicle accident (MVA) has sustained blunt nonpenetrating trauma to the chest. Upon arrival in the emergency department, the nurse observes asymmetrical chest rise. Which action(s) by the nurse indicate(s) an understanding of the presenting symptom?

I. Preparation for placement of a chest drain.
II. Assessment of oxygenation.
III. Administration of pain medication.
IV. Collection of a detailed medical history.

a. Choices II and III
b. Choices II, III, and IV
c. Choices I and III
d. Choices I and II

21. Which of the following is critical for a medical facility to establish prior to a natural disaster ever occurring?

a. A hurricane evacuation plan
b. A temporary morgue
c. Interim chain of command
d. Storage of extra PPE

22. Failed intubation is indicative of which of the following emergency conditions?

a. Medical suction
b. A heart attack
c. A blown vein
d. A difficult airway

23. Lia, a nurse, is working a night shift in the emergency department. A patient is brought in by his wife, who reports that the patient fell and bumped his head on a sharp coffee table. Although the patient is walking adequately when supported, he appears confused and his speech is slurred. He is unable to move one arm and reports sharp pain on one side of his head. Suddenly, he begins to vomit. What issue should this patient be examined for immediately upon intake?

a. Intracerebral hemorrhage
b. Meningitis
c. A bone fracture
d. Dementia

Professional Accountabilities

1. Under what circumstance should the circulator speak up if they feel a team member's behavior undermines a culture of safety?

a. At any time, regardless of the team member's role
b. Only if it is a fellow nursing team member
c. Only if it involves a fellow nursing team member or scrub technician
d. Only if it does not involve the primary surgeon

2. The scrub technician informs the nurse that they believe a nonsterile team member brushed against the edge of the sterile table. What should the circulator do next?
   a. Ask if other team members witnessed the activity.
   b. Ask the surgeon how they would like to proceed.
   c. Assume the edge of the sterile table has been contaminated.
   d. Only assume it was contaminated if they saw the reported activity.

3. When should nurses participate in professional development activities?
   a. Only if required by the facility
   b. Whenever possible
   c. Only when compensated
   d. Whenever a JCAHO audit is suspected

4. The surgeon asks to use a piece of equipment that the circulator and scrub nurse have not been trained on. Which of the following actions is most appropriate?
   a. Refuse to open the piece of equipment onto the sterile field.
   b. Ask the charge nurse if the equipment representative is available for assistance.
   c. Assume the surgeon will know how to assemble and operate the equipment.
   d. Open the equipment without mentioning that the staff has not been trained to use the equipment.

5. Which of the following statements is true in the event of an incorrect count involving a very small needle?
   a. An x-ray should always be taken.
   b. The surgeon does not need to be informed.
   c. The documentation does not need to reflect that the count was incorrect.
   d. The staff should search for the needle even though it is very small.

6. When should adverse events that occur at the end of the nurse's shift be reported?
   a. The following day
   b. As soon as reasonably possible
   c. Only if there is litigation
   d. Only if it was a never event and in full detail in the patient's medical record

7. At minimum, which sets of standards and guidelines should all perioperative nurses familiarize themselves with?
   a. FDA and EPA standards and guidelines
   b. OSHA and ANA standards and guidelines, in addition to the guidelines of the state in which they work
   c. HHS and DPH standards and guidelines for the country and state in which they work
   d. CDC standards and guidelines

8. Patient safety, patient physiological response to surgical procedures, patient and family behavioral responses to surgical procedures, and the health system where the surgery is performed are the four focal domains of patient-centered care as established by which reputable organization?
   a. The CDC
   b. The AORN
   c. Mayo Clinic
   d. Johns Hopkins University

9. Janna and Maya are two nurses scrubbing in for a surgical case. Janna is a nurse anesthetist, and Maya is a surgical nurse practitioner. Janna casually mentions that she hopes their current case is more straightforward than the complex case they had this morning, as she is still feeling a bit drained from it. Maya has been a nurse practitioner in this surgery unit for almost a decade and tells Janna she can oversee her responsibilities if needed. How should Janna respond?
   a. Janna should not let Maya take over her responsibilities, as they are outside of Maya's scope of responsibility.
   b. Janna should thank Maya, and let the team know that they can ask either her or Maya any relevant questions or take over any related tasks.
   c. Janna doesn't need to respond in any particular way, but Maya should report Janna to the nurse manager for feeling fatigued after one case.
   d. Janna should utilize Maya as a backup resource during the case if she feels unable to focus at any point.

10. Service-line management, charge nurse, managing nurse, and information technology analyst are all examples of what?
   a. Professional growth opportunities for perioperative nurses
   b. Internship opportunities for first-year nursing students
   c. Tasks only medical doctors should be responsible for
   d. Virtual healthcare roles

11. Douglas is a nurse in a dermatology clinic. He notices during some surgical procedures that the hand sanitization station is in a difficult location for many team members to reach, and that waiting while everyone washes and sanitizes their hands before placing their gloves on before a procedure can take up to 45 minutes. The clinic is often delayed during their daily schedule. Douglas speaks with the clinic manager and proposes moving the hand sanitization station to a more common area. After a month, he documents that the overall clinic delay time has decreased by approximately 20 minutes per day. What is this an example of?
   a. WHO global sanitization efforts
   b. JHCO regulations
   c. Quality improvement
   d. A common dermatology clinic issue

12. Hanna is a new perioperative nurse who sees a device package that she believes isn't sterile. Hanna's colleague, Diana, says she retrieved the device package and has no reason to believe that its sterilization was compromised. What should the surgical team do in this case?

a. Give Diana the benefit, due to her seniority
b. Send both nurses to HR for intrapersonal relationship counseling
c. Ask Hanna to provide concrete reasoning as to why she believes the package sterility was compromised
d. Discard the device in question and use a new package

13. Which of the following is a framework in continuous quality improvement that can be used by frontline workers to test changes in the nursing environment?

a. PDSA cycle
b. DMAIC method
c. Value-stream mapping
d. Lean

14. Which of the following is likely outside of the nursing scope of practice for a registered nurse?

a. Delegating nursing responsibilities
b. Inserting catheters
c. Prescribing and administering medications
d. Monitoring patient vitals

15. Joan is a registered nurse who works at a university health center. One of her main job duties is to recruit students to participate in a stress study. Students who are eligible and provide informed consent to participate work with Joan over a course of three months. During this time, Joan takes a weekly blood sample and analyzes it for various elements, including insulin and cortisol levels. She also provides a weekly mindfulness intervention and has a student assistant who collects self-reported questionnaires from each participant. Joan and her assistant provide all data to the principal investigator who hired Joan. What type of occupational position within nursing does Joan likely hold?

a. Doctoral candidate
b. Clinical research nurse
c. Assistant teaching professor
d. Nurse administrator

Answer Explanations

Pre/Postoperative Patient Assessment and Diagnosis

1. C: The diagnostic procedures performed depend on the planned surgical procedure, patient's history, risk factors, and best practice standards. These can be done in various settings, such as physician's office, laboratory, outpatient clinic, or hospital. They can be completed up to a few months prior to the procedure, depending on the test. Diagnostic procedures are based on individualized patient assessment information, not specifically on the type of procedure to be performed.

2. D: The surgeon and anesthesiologist need to know if the report is missing, as they will be reviewing it to ensure the patient is cleared from a cardiac standpoint for surgery. The nurse should not assume the patient did not undergo the test because the results are not in the chart. Additionally, asking the patient why it wasn't done is accusatory and unprofessional. The nurse cannot assume the case will be canceled and should not allow the patient to eat unless diet orders are received. Determining the patient does not need the cardiac catheterization is outside the nurse's scope of practice.

3. D: The patient interview adds subjective assessment data to the nurse's findings. Auscultation, palpation, and percussion yield objective assessment data.

4. B: Screening tools are standards of care and are utilized in the preoperative assessment. Focused assessments may be conducted based on initial assessment findings. The nurse implements plans based on abnormal screening tool findings. The screening tool itself does not provide abnormal lab values. The nurse should consult with interdisciplinary teams, when indicated. The use of screening tools does not decrease the likelihood of using interdisciplinary teams.

5. A: Anxiety related to the disease process is the most appropriate nursing diagnosis based on the given information. The risk of hypothermia is not increased based on her age or length of surgery. Dehydration, although a potential risk, is not the most likely situation for this patient. The surgical procedure is short, and risk of impaired skin integrity based on the length of procedure is not a high priority for this patient.

6. C: In this situation, implementation of the preoperative plan of care interventions begins during the preoperative phase of care. This patient's nursing diagnosis is anxiety related to the disease process. To be most effective, the nurse begins implementing anxiety-reduction measures in the preoperative period. Waiting until the later phases of care will not ease the patient's anxiety and fears regarding the disease process.

7. C: During the patient identity phase, the nurse uses two patient identifiers—typically, the patient's name and date of birth. The patient's medical record number may also be used, but not the social security number. Verification of the surgical site is not part of the patient identification process.

8. B: Whenever possible, the patient should be involved in the surgical site-marking process. The site should not be marked with an "X," as this can be ambiguous. The site should be marked with either "yes" or the surgeon's initials. Surgical site marking should be visible after draping.

9. D: The patient who is oriented to name only is not competent to make informed decisions in the consent process. Patients under eighteen years of age (not twenty years of age) are considered minors. A flat affect does not indicate lack of decision-making ability. Narcotic medications taken the day before surgery do not affect decision-making ability in the consent process.

10. D: Emergent procedures are the only exception when it comes to requirement of consent prior to procedure. Consent for pediatric patients is given by the patient's parent or legal guardian. Surgery is a type of invasive procedure. Routine procedures fall under Universal Protocol guidelines.

11. C: Advance directives address the patient's do not resuscitate (DNR) status. Religious support is an aspect of culturally competent care. Postoperative pain management is not part of the Advance Directives document.

12. D: If a patient is entering surgery with a DNR order of anything other than full code, this must be communicated to the entire surgical team and documented in the medical record.

13. B: The objective assessment is the data collection piece (lab values, vital signs, physical assessment, etc.). Implementation occurs after the nursing diagnoses are made. Nursing diagnoses are formulated based on assessment data. During evaluation, the nurse identifies whether or not specific goals were met.

14. C: The final phase of the nursing process is evaluation; however, evaluation happens across the continuum of the nursing process, not just at the end. The nurse frequently evaluates the effectiveness of care plans, adjusts as necessary, and reevaluates. Data is collected during the assessment phase. Nursing diagnoses are formulated in the diagnosis phase. The implementation phase often begins with educating the patient on expected outcomes.

15. A: The next step the nurse should take is notifying the surgeon and anesthesiologist of the patient remaining on blood thinners, as this will affect the decision to proceed with the surgery or not. Asking the patient why they remained on the medication does not change the outcome. Continuing with the medication reconciliation process may or may not need to happen, as the surgery may be canceled. Assessing the patient's education level is not an immediate priority.

16. B: Use of recreational drugs should be included in the medication reconciliation process. The prescriber of the current medications is not relevant during the reconciliation process. Prescription medication, as well as over-the-counter medications, supplements, and vitamins, should be noted. The patient's preferred pharmacy is not included in the medication reconciliation process.

17. B: The use of electronic medical records (EMRs) is considered best practice and provides rapid access to patient information by the entire health care team. Paper documentation is not as readily available and can only be in one location at a time. Blended and compartmentalized documentation are not identified as types of health care documentation.

18. D: In preparing the patient for the operative phase of care, the preoperative nurse completes tasks to promote optimal patient outcomes and patient safety. Best use of time and resources, decreased turnover time between surgical cases, and cost-effectiveness do not trump patient safety and optimal patient outcomes.

19. B: The physical assessment includes documentation of impaired skin integrity, mobility limitations, and presence of body piercings or implanted foreign objects. Planning, intervention, and diagnosis phases do not specifically address the collection of data.

20. B: Hair removal occurs during the immediate preoperative period, after the preoperative assessment, intake of patient history, medication reconciliation, consent process, and patient verbalization of plan of care. Review of cardiac catheterization results, pulmonary function testing, and consideration of alternative treatment options occurs prior to the decision to proceed with surgery.

21. B: This information falls under protected health information, meaning it's protected under HIPAA and cannot be freely shared, even with immediate family members (unless the patient is a minor). Healthcare personnel should be mindful not to openly discuss these unless necessary for the patient's care.

22. A: The World Health Organization (WHO) created the Surgical Safety Checklist with the intention to promote patient safety and to improve documentation standards. The remaining answers are partially correct. The checklists aim to reduce the risk for complications before, during, and after surgery.

23. B: A checklist can only be useful if all active members work together to use it at the same time; otherwise, it cannot produce standardized results. Aesthetically pleasing checklists can be nice but aren't necessary. Checklist tasks should always be repeatable and reliable; therefore, diverse tasks would make a poor checklist. A checklist doesn't need a global presence to be a reliable tool; it simply needs to be accepted by the organization and staff where it's being used as a quality tool.

24. C: Patients respond favorably to positive intrapersonal communication between their attending nurses and physicians. The other options may be nice for patients, but studies indicate that nurse and physician relationships have the most impact on a patient's overall experience.

25. C: Choice *C* represents an accurate understanding of the first step, verification, as an accurate medication history is obtained. Choice *A* and Choice *B* represent a misunderstanding by the licensed practical nurse (LPN), as these actions align with clarification, which is the second step of the medication reconciliation process. Choice *D* aligns with the third and final step of the process, reconciliation.

26. B: When illicit drugs are discovered during the physical assessment of a patient, the nurses must page the nursing supervisor to elevate the concern, so Choice *B* is correct. The supervisor will then remove the drugs from the unit with security personnel and they will be destroyed. It would not be appropriate for the nurses to send the drugs home with the patient's spouse, Choice *C*, or plan to return them to the patient at discharge, Choice *D*. Additionally, contacting police to report this finding as a crime would not be legally supported, Choice *A*.

27. B: Auscultation, Choice *B,* is the second step of an abdominal physical assessment. The nurse should first perform Choice *C*, inspection, then Choice *B*, auscultation, followed by Choice *A*, percussion, and finally Choice *D*, palpation. This sequence of techniques is unique to an abdominal physical assessment to promote accuracy in findings by not interfering with the results.

28. C: Palpate, Choice *C,* represents the second step of a respiratory physical assessment. The nurse should first perform Choice *A*, inspect, then Choice *C*, palpate, followed by Choice *B*, percuss, and finally Choice *D*, auscultate. This sequence of techniques is standard for physical assessments—except when performing an abdominal assessment—to promote accuracy in findings.

29. D: The patient's preferences, values, and beliefs, as well as indication of a surrogate decision maker, are all included in advance directives.

30. C: Medication titration, Choice *C,* involves titrating the dosage to reach a therapeutic level, as it encourages careful consideration to achieve the maximum benefit without adverse reaction. Medication compliance, Choice *A,* involves patient agreement and fulfillment of medication intake. Medication reconciliation, Choice *B,* describes the process of creating a list of medications taken. Medication administration, Choice *D,* involves the practice of delivering medication for intake.

31. B: Reliable and Joint Commission recommended patient identifiers should be used at all patient handoffs and when using any patient specimen samples to ensure that the care provider is treating the correct patient. This ensures the patient's safety and quality of medical care, and also reduces the risk of liability and wasted resources for the care provider. Full name and date of birth are two reliable patient identifiers that can be used to confirm patient identity.

Other options recommended by the Joint Commission as reliable patient identifiers include Social Security number, electronic medical number, address, or government-issued photo identification. The facility and treatment protocol information are important pieces of information, and are generally sent over by the initial care team. This information is not useful until the patient has been accurately identified, and as multiple patients can arrive from the same facility with similar conditions, these are not reliable or safe patient identifiers.

Choice *A* can be eliminated. Patient insurance information and weight are not reliable patient identifiers and likely would not be taken immediately upon receiving a transfer, so Choice *C* is incorrect. While date of birth is a reliable patient identifier, patients should not be charged with confirming prior procedures and medications upon a transfer. This is also not a reliable method of identifying a patient. Therefore, Choice *D* can be eliminated.

32. D: Multi-modal pain management therapies, in which various non-opioid pain medications are used to manage a patient's pain, have been linked with reduced need for opioids and reduced adverse effects (such as dependency and withdrawal symptoms) associated with opioid use. As opioid use is an epidemic linked with severe health outcomes and patient issues, reducing its use and adverse effects is a great benefit. Multi-modal pain therapies tailor the medications a patient needs to manage their pain, since pain tolerance is highly subjective. Therefore, these therapies do not standardize treatment and instead develop a plan that is best for an individual patient, eliminating Choice *A*. They also often require multiple types of medications rather than a single medication, so Choice *B* can be eliminated. This type of therapy does not necessarily reduce insurance costs, although it may in instances where the patient has better overall health outcomes as a result of effective pain management. Therefore, Choice *C* is incorrect.

33. A: Advance directives provide instructions for medical providers and family members to follow in case a patient is unable to make decisions on their own (e.g., during an emergency surgery). An advance directive allows the patient to document their own wishes regarding the care they receive and is considered a legally binding document. A last will and testament can provide information for what a patient may wish for upon death (e.g., cremation versus burial) as well as designations regarding their estate, but does not usually have information specific to medical procedures and outcomes. Choice *B* can be eliminated. Similarly, beneficiaries are the people designated to receive assets due a patient's death and are not relevant to procedures that should be followed during a medical event. Therefore,

Choice *C* is incorrect. A primary policyholder document refers to paperwork people receive outlining provisions of policies they own, such as insurance policies. This question is not relevant for Liam's situation, so Choice *D* can be eliminated.

Individualized Plan of Care Development and Expected Outcomes

1. A: CMS is the government administrator of Medicare and Medicaid, and it is responsible for the financial regulation of them. Notably, CMS imposes financial fees on health care organizations for negative patient outcomes, including pressure ulcers (stage III and IV), falls, surgical site infection (SSI), retained foreign objects, wrong site surgery, and deep vein thrombosis (DVT). TJC, IOM, and WHO do not directly impose financial fees on organizations based on negative patient outcomes.

2. C: Situational factors include fatigue, being under the influence of drugs or alcohol, stress, and distractions such as background noise and conversations. Skill-based behavior errors generally occur when the nurse fails to monitor the actions being performed or when the nurse's attention is diverted. Knowledge-based performance errors are those involving perception, inference, interpretation, and judgment.

3. C: HIPAA protects patient rights around confidentiality, release of medical information, and privacy. A Patient Bill of Rights is a document that communicates the patient's rights and responsibilities when it comes to health care. The WHO Surgical Safety Checklist was launched by the WHO in 2004 to examine patient safety in the settings of primary and acute care. TJC's National Patient Safety Goals (NPSGs) are formulated from reviewing best practice guidelines, as well as sentinel events.

4. C: If the patient is prescribed medications, it is the patient's responsibility to keep medications to self only, not allowing others access to them. The patient is responsible for disclosing use of all medications to the health care team, including over-the-counter medications. The patient may use more than one pharmacy at a time. The patient is not responsible for knowing all the pharmacological effects and possible adverse reactions of medication combinations; they should be educated on this by the pharmacist and prescribing physician.

5. D: Regulatory bodies such as TJC and CMS clearly identify patient education as a need that must be fulfilled in order to promote optimal patient outcomes. While holistic care, discharge planning, and culturally based care are important aspects of nursing, these are not identified by TJC and CMS as ones that must be fulfilled in order to promote optimal patient outcomes.

6. B: Liability means to be responsible to or under obligation, and negligence is defined as the failure to exercise the standard of care that a reasonably prudent person would exercise under similar conditions. Each state board of nursing has a Nursing Practice Act that sets the standards of care a nurse is expected to maintain in practice.

7. A: Each state board of nursing has a Nursing Practice Act that sets the standards of care a nurse is expected to maintain in practice. All fifty states do not require nurses to maintain a minimum number of CEUs. Policies and procedures vary from institutions within each state. Nursing Practice Acts are regulated by states, not federally.

8. D: Geographical community resources include public libraries and government offices. Institutional resources include tuition reimbursement, employee assistance programs (EAPs), and other health care professionals. Local and demographical resources are not specific types of resources for patient/family education.

9. A: CMS withholds reimbursement to institutions and providers if a patient is readmitted to the hospital within thirty days of discharge if the readmission is related to the same problem causing the initial hospitalization. Complications such as extended ventilator run and postoperative atrial fibrillation are not cause for withholding reimbursement to providers. Observing the patient with a history of renal failure for an extra day in the hospital does not warrant withholding reimbursement from CMS.

10. A: EHRs have been shown to reduce (and even prevent) medical errors due to misinterpretation of handwriting. EHRs also allow built-in systems designed to prevent treatment errors. EHRs do not relate to the time spent researching a disease process.

11. D: Hand hygiene is the gold standard for preventing disease transmission. Antibiotic prophylaxis, decreasing surface contaminants, and screening visitors for communicable disease are ways to decrease nosocomial infections, but they are not recognized as the gold standard.

12. B: Transmission-based precautions are classified in three ways: contact, droplet, and airborne. Surface precautions are not an example of transmission-based precautions.

13. B: Tasks related to current Surgical Care Improvement Project (SCIP) measures are implemented by the surgical team preoperatively. These include preoperative antibiotic prophylaxis, administration of beta-blocker drugs in certain patients, and application of antiembolism stockings or compression devices. Verification of blood product availability is not an SCIP measure.

14. C: Age-specific needs are incorporated in the care plan as needed. This may include providing a tangible comfort item, such as a blanket or toy. Providing an interpreter or chaplain demonstrates culturally competent care. Discussing postoperative pain management is not age-specific care.

15. D: Each of these items are content that should be included with discharge instructions provided to the patient or family.

16. A: Postoperative follow-up calls are an opportunity for perioperative staff to assess recovery of the patient, address questions, provide reinforcement education, and identify any discrepancies that could have a negative impact on the patient's postoperative period. Patient satisfaction calls are not typically conducted by the perioperative staff.

17. D: I-PASS is a structured handoff used to improve quality of care by defining the points of information that should be communicated any time a patient's care is transferred to another provider (e.g., new facility, shift changes). It stands for Illness severity, Patient information, Action list, Situational awareness, and Synthesis by receiver. MRSA stands for Methicillin-resistant Staphylococcus Aureus, a bacteria group that is resistant to antibiotic treatments. It does not have anything to do with medical handoffs, so Choice *A* can be eliminated. STAR is not an acronym used in medical care, although medical facilities can receive a quality STAR rating for patient outcomes. It is not related to provider handoffs, so Choice *B* can be eliminated. SBAR stands for Situation, Background, Assessment, Recommendation and has previously been used in handoff contexts; however, it has been generally replaced with I-PASS. I-PASS is considered to be more comprehensive in handoff situations and demonstrates a higher efficacy in patient care and safety, while SBAR may be used more often in emergency situations. Therefore, Choice *C* can be eliminated.

18. B: Older elementary-school-aged patients and pre-adolescent patients are in a developmental stage where they tend to take most pieces of information literally. If told that they will be "put to sleep" for a surgery, they are likely to believe that they may wake up during the procedure, similar to how they would wake up from actual sleep. Therefore, providers should explain the anesthesia process in a way that makes sense to a mind in this stage of development to avoid any unnecessary or irrational fear. While any parent is likely to feel anxious when their child is undergoing surgery, studies indicate that parental anxiety is highest when the patient is six months of age or younger; therefore, Choice *A* can be eliminated. Studies also indicate that separation anxiety in pediatric surgical patients decreases significantly after age eight, so Choice *C* is incorrect; it is not the most likely event that a nine-year-old patient would experience. Infants are the pediatric age group most likely to not be aware of their surroundings during surgical procedures due to their early developmental stage. The average nine-year-old patient would be well aware that a medical event was occurring, so Choice *D* is incorrect.

Intraoperative Activities

1. C: The CDC reports healthcare providers clean their hands less than one half of the times they should. Hand hygiene in the form of surgical scrubbing is required prior to donning sterile gloves in the perioperative environment. A two-minute hand wash after leaving a patient care area is not supported by evidence. Hand washing can reduce the spread of MDROs.

2. B: The insertion of a medication port does not require a long operative time, does not involve the genitourinary tract, does not pose risk of urine entering the sterile field, does not require intraoperative urinary output monitoring, and does not necessitate core temperature monitoring. Therefore, this patient is not a candidate for perioperative urinary catheter insertion. The patient undergoing cardiac transplant requires intraoperative urinary output and core temperature monitoring. A bladder resection involves the genitourinary tract. A femoral-popliteal revascularization surgery requires the groin to be in the surgical field, so the absence of a urinary catheter poses the risk of urine entering the sterile field.

3. A: Since the package containing the laparotomy sponges is compromised, the contents of the package are contaminated. Once the contaminated laparotomy sponges enter the basin, the entire contents of the basin are considered contaminated and must be discarded. Since sterile items must be contained in a sterile field, and the sterile field was broken when the contaminated sponges entered the basin, the entire basin is considered contaminated, and removing select pieces and keeping others is not recommended. The sterile field is established once sterile supplies are opened in the room, regardless of whether a patient is present or not. Since the situation can be rectified prior to touching the patient, this case is not Class III (contaminated).

4. A: The surgical gown sterile zones are the front (chest level to level of sterile field) and at the sleeves from two inches above the elbow to sleeve cuff. The back of the surgical gown is not considered sterile.

5. C: Nonsterile persons should not walk in between two sterile fields. Once skin prep begins, the patient is considered to be in a sterile field. Nonsterile team members must remain a minimum of twelve inches away from the sterile field. Exiting the room into the sterile hallway to obtain necessary equipment or supplies is recommended practice. Nonsterile objects, including the arm of a nonsterile person, should not reach over the sterile field.

6. B: Skin prep inhibits rebound microorganism growth on the skin. Skin prep is not intended to sterilize the skin. Skin prep decreases the number of resident microorganisms. Removing visible soil and debris should be done first, not last. The order of the three objectives is as follows: remove the soil, debris, and transient microorganisms from the skin surface; reduce the number of resident microorganisms on the skin; and inhibit rebound microorganism growth on the skin.

7. B: ChloraPrep is an alcohol-based chlorhexidine gluconate solution. Alcohol-based solutions are contraindicated on open wounds. ChloraPrep is safe for the patient with a povidone iodine allergy. It is indicated for use on intact skin areas (such as left groin and chest).

8. D: As a result of the report, the IOM instituted six recommendations for improvement of patient safety: healthcare that is safe, effective, patient-centered, timely, efficient, and equitable. The use of the WHO surgical safety checklist is considered best practice. The report findings indicate patient safety is influenced by multiple factors in concert with each other, not one primary factor. Addressing the objectives of the report requires action from all parties involved with patient care, from direct patient caregivers to hospital administrators.

9. A: Establishing a no-distraction zone in medication preparation areas minimizes the risk of medication error. Air exchanges should not be decreased past the set requirement, because this creates an infection control hazard. Traffic patterns should be kept to a minimum but cannot be eliminated. The use of smoke evacuators is considered best practice for personnel safety and should not be eliminated.

10. B: Since perioperative personnel are at risk for chemical and biohazard exposure, introduction to HAZMAT information should be done at the beginning of employment. Presenting the education should not be delayed for six months. Additionally, it should not only be introduced and reviewed during annual mandatory education. The HAZMAT manual should be referenced in the event of exposure as well as beginning of employment.

11. C: Ergonomics is the science of matching the physical requirements of a job to the physical abilities of the worker. Body mechanics refers to how the body moves during activities of daily living. Neither physical dexterity nor foundational movement is related to matching physical requirements of a job to the physical abilities of the worker.

12. C: Using SPM equipment during lateral transfers is an evidence-based practice in preventing associate injury. Applying a safety strap does not necessitate the use of SPM. Rotating the bed and raising the head of the bed are both done remotely and do not require lifting or physical effort beyond pressing a button on the bed's remote control.

13. A: If the procedure is one hour or greater in duration, thermoregulation measures should be taken to prevent hypothermia.

14. B: If the patient indicates a history of MH or a family history of difficulty with anesthesia, the perioperative team should be prepared for MH crisis and discuss this risk with the entire perioperative team. Elevated serum potassium level, presence of first-degree atrioventricular heart block, and postoperative nausea and vomiting are not indicators of MH risk.

15. A: The perioperative nurse, anesthesiologist, and surgeon work together in positioning the patient for surgery. Although responsibility lies with the nurse, anesthesiologist, and surgeon, the surgical technologist may participate under the guidance of these team members.

16. C: In the supine position, the patient lies on their back with legs on the bed. This is the routine position for most abdominal, open heart, and lower extremity procedures. In lithotomy position, the patient's legs are in stirrups; this is indicated for gynecological, urology, and colorectal procedures. In left lateral position, the patient lies on their left side with right side up.

17. D: Each elbow should be padded prior to tucking to protect the ulnar nerve. The vagus, phrenic, and sciatic nerves are not affected during tucking of the arms.

18. D: Patient conditions known to adversely influence the body's wound healing capability are malnutrition, hyperglycemia, obesity, smoking, and respiratory compromise. Mrs. Johnson has two of these conditions.

19. C: Delayed primary closure is often used in the case of compartment syndrome, where swelling is highly anticipated. Primary union is the preferred method for wound healing. Collagen fibers connect together during the final phase (remodeling phase) of wound healing. Genitourinary cases are not an indication for delayed wound closure.

20. A: Since the procedure involved the prostate, which is part of the genitourinary tract, it is a Class II (clean contaminated) case.

21. B: In a case with major break in sterile technique, it becomes a Class III (contaminated) case. Class IV (dirty/infected) indicates microorganisms that can cause SSI are present before the time of surgery. Major break in sterile technique eliminates Class I (clean) and Class II (clean contaminated).

22. A: SSI may be improperly labeled as "hospital-acquired" if the surgical wound class is not properly identified. This label can result in CMS's withholding reimbursement to the healthcare facility and providers. TJC does not penalize hospitals for performing Class IV surgeries. Incorrect documentation of surgical wound class does not directly affect patient's discharge timeframe. Surgical wound class predicts the patient's risk for developing SSI, not postoperative hemorrhage.

23. A: The patient with severe systemic disease that is not incapacitating, such as uncontrolled diabetes or end stage renal disease, is an ASA III. ASA IV indicates severe systemic disease that is a constant threat to life (i.e., recent MI, cardiac ischemia). ASA V describes the patient who is near death and not expected to survive without the operation. The ASA VI patient is one who has been declared brain dead and is being kept alive for the purposes of organ harvesting.

24. C: Regional anesthesia is achieved when local anesthetic is injected along a nerve pathway. Types of regional anesthesia are spinal, epidural, and Bier block. General anesthesia dramatically alters the patient's mental status and consists of amnesia, analgesia, and muscle relaxation. Local anesthetic involves injecting medication such as bupivacaine or lidocaine at the surgical site, not along a nerve pathway. In MAC, the patient receives local anesthetic along with sedation and analgesia.

25. D: During the preoperative phase, the nurse and anesthesiologist review the patient's medical history and develop the pain management plan. The plan is carried out through the intraoperative and postoperative phases. The suboperative phase does not exist.

26. D: Fentanyl, hydromorphone, and morphine are opioid analgesics commonly used in the perioperative environment. Ketorolac is an anti-inflammatory medication. Succinylcholine is a paralytic, and lidocaine is a local anesthetic.

27. B: Perioperative medication administration documentation includes the name, dose, route, and time of medication. Documentation of the medication expiration date is not required.

28. A: If the person discovering the narcotic discrepancy is unable to resolve it, the issue is immediately turned over to security and/or pharmacy, depending on healthcare institution policy. The discrepancy should not be ignored. Although education may be a good idea, it is not the immediate next step. Retrieving hydromorphone from another Pyxis unit will not resolve the discrepancy.

29. D: Surgical scissors can be used after skin incision to dissect tissue for exposure to the surgical area. Clamps have "teeth" that come together when the clamp is engaged. Graspers are designed to hold or grasp tissue and provide traction away from the surgical area. Scopes are used for visualization in minimally invasive procedures.

30. A: A pneumatic tourniquet is used in vascular and orthopedic procedures to reduce blood flow at the surgical site during critical points of the operation. X-ray detectable gauze is designed to absorb fluid in small amounts. A surgical safety knife blade is used during skin incision or incision into blood vessels. Ventilator circuits are part of the anesthesia machine setup and provide a conduit for delivering oxygen to the patient.

31. C: A surgical implant refers to an item intentionally placed inside the body during surgery that will remain in place permanently, or for a specified time frame, generally longer than twenty-one days. A mechanical heart valve is a permanent implant. A nasogastric tube, intravenous catheter, and indwelling urinary catheter are neither permanent, nor designed to remain in place for longer than twenty-one days.

32. A: Unless deemed unsafe, the surgical implant should be removed in the case of infection resulting from the implant. Antibiotic prophylaxis does not alter the integrity of the implant. Documentation does not include the implant's cost. Biological sources often include human donors.

33. B: A retained surgical item can ultimately result in patient death. While a retained surgical item may increase the length of stay, cost of care, or risk of infection, patient mortality is the worst possible outcome.

34. B: Surgical counts are performed prior to skin incision, at the beginning of closure of body cavity or first tissue layer, and during skin closure. They are not performed upon arrival at the recovery unit.

35. A: The surgical count may be omitted in the case of an emergency. A ruptured abdominal aortic aneurysm and blood pressure of 50/30 indicates an emergency. Left arm pain with stable vital signs is not an emergency. The surgeon's being in a hurry and the patient with a "no code" status are not valid reasons for omitting surgical counts.

36. B: A surgical specimen is body fluid or tissue removed from the body during the surgical procedure. Of these choices, the portion of left lower lobe of lung is the only item that fits the surgical specimen definition.

37. D: If a foreign body is discovered during surgery, it should be labeled as "foreign body" or "retained surgical item" and sent to pathology for identification. The item should not be referred to as a "thumb tack," since it is a foreign body.

38. D: Patient body fluids and excreta are biological hazards. Cytotoxic and chemotherapy medications are chemical hazards. Laser and ultraviolet radiation are radiological hazards. Autoclaves and carbon dioxide tanks are examples of potential physical hazards.

39. D: Perioperative hazards should be discussed at the beginning of employment in the perioperative environment. Education should also be provided on an ongoing basis, according to healthcare facility policy.

40. B: Smoke plumes can potentially contain hazardous gases, including hydrogen cyanide and formaldehyde. They can also contain viruses and live biological material. According to researchers, smoke plumes can increase cancer risk for perioperative team members by way of inhaling the surgical smoke. Smoke plumes are not a result of exhaled anesthetic gases. They do not set off an operating room's sprinkler system. They do not decrease visibility of the surgical site.

41. A: AORN recommends the use of smoke evacuators in all cases with the use of electrosurgical cautery or laser, regardless of the length of the surgical case. AORN recommendations for smoke evacuator use are not based on patient diagnosis or presence of communicable disease.

42. B: If the patient condition warrants temperature adjustment below the range outlined in policy, such as in cardiopulmonary circulatory arrest, the surgeon documents the temperature adjustment and rationale in the patient's medical record. The surgeon's comfort level is not a rationale for decreasing the room temperature below outlined parameters. Temperatures below acceptable range (outlined in policy) can lead to hypothermia, which increases risk for SSI. The surgical time is not a factor in adjusting room temperature outside of acceptable range.

43. B: Humidity levels in the operating room are generally kept between twenty and sixty percent.

44. C: One way to control noise levels is to avoid unnecessary conversations and keep voices low. Muffling devices for equipment are not used. Silencing the telephone is not an evidence-based practice and may contribute to delays in critical communication. Although room traffic should be kept to a minimum, it cannot be eliminated.

45. A: For patients receiving anticoagulation therapy, protime/international ratio (PT/INR) and partial thromboplastin time (PTT) are tested to determine need for anticoagulation reversal agents. Blood urea nitrogen (BUN) is a lab test of kidney function. Hemoglobin and hematocrit levels indicate blood volume status.

46. C: Intraoperative cell salvage is widely used in cases in which a high amount of blood loss is anticipated. Cryoprecipitate transfusion occurs when fibrinogen levels are low in patients with active bleeding. Platelet therapy is done when patients have low platelet levels preoperatively or during surgery, if the patient is actively bleeding. The use of ABO uncrossmatched blood happens in emergent situations in which the patient has not been ABO crossmatched.

47. C: TJC and CMS mandate the manufacturer's instructions for use to be present in areas using the equipment. The WHO equipment safety checklist, FDA equipment manual, and SCIP equipment log are not items used in operating rooms.

48. A: It is important for care providers to only use the equipment per manufacturer guidelines, since these guidelines are the ones tested and approved as safe for patient use by the FDA. If a safety concern regarding the equipment arises, the FDA recalls the product until the safety issue is resolved. TJC, CMS, and OSHA are not in charge of regulating medical equipment safety.

49. D: If a piece of surgical equipment poses a potential fire hazard, the IFU contains information stating the type of fire extinguisher to have available. The type of intravenous fluids, warming blanket, and x-ray detectable gauze used on the patient are not related to the potential fire hazard.

50. B: The RNFA is not the individual performing the procedure, and therefore, should not perform the surgical time-out. A surgery resident may make the initial incision under the appropriate supervision, and a surgical fellow can close the incision. X-ray technicians may be required for certain procedures where x-ray is needed intraoperatively.

51. B: Many facilities have instituted successful recycling programs for certain types of approved materials, but these programs must be implemented with a goal of eliminating the possibility of infection or contamination. It is not possible to recycle all types of materials, and recycling programs should not be based on a surgeon's personal preferences.

52. D: Product selection should be completed by the interdisciplinary surgical team, and it should take into account the cost of the item to the facility, what the surgeon prefers, and what products have been proven effective in the market. A surgeon preference should not be the sole factor in the product selection because many off-brand materials are equally effective.

53. B: In some cases, it may be beneficial to the patient to have a family member in the OR before induction to ease the patient's anxiety. However, the circulator should always be aware of the potential for visitors to compromise the sterile field, and it is not required to accommodate every request to escort the patient into the OR. The circulator should closely supervise any family members into the OR and have them escorted out of the OR after the patient is asleep.

54. A: Terminal cleaning should ideally be completed daily and at the end of the cases for the day. The equipment should either be removed from the room or moved so that the staff can ensure there is no debris under the equipment. Terminal cleaning is not required in between cases or after procedures on patients on isolation precautions. Further, to reduce the potential impact to morning on-time starts, terminal cleaning should be completed at the end of the day rather than before the first case of the day.

55. C: The temperature indicator on an implant should be examined both when the tissue arrives at the facility and before the tissue is implanted. When the tissue arrives at the facility, the indicator should be inspected to ensure that the tissue was not compromised during transport. Prior to implanting the tissue, the indicator should be inspected to confirm that the tissue was not compromised while being stored at the facility. However, it is not required that the indicator is inspected daily.

56. B: N-95 masks should be used when caring for a patient with tuberculosis to prevent transmission. When caring for a patient with MRSA, VRE, or *C. difficile,* the staff should implement contact precautions and ensure that they are wearing gloves and gowns when there is a potential for patient contact. However, standard masks are acceptable when interacting with these patients.

57. D: For essential equipment like a microscope, the circulator should ensure that the equipment should be available at the required time before bringing the patient back to the OR. If the equipment is not likely to be available when needed, the staff may need to delay the case to ensure the equipment will be available when needed.

58. C: Product evaluation and selection should continually take place because new products and alternatives are constantly entering the market. While the opinions and preferences of the primary surgeon are very important, the evaluation and selection should involve the entire team to ensure the most cost-effective product is selected.

59. A: Vendor supervision is always required because it ensures maintained integrity of the sterile field and optimal care for the patient. Vendors are required to undergo training and certification; however, the circulator should constantly monitor their actions to prevent accidental contamination. Further, vendors have the potential to be a distraction to the surgical team, and the circulator should intervene if the vendor is acting inappropriately.

60. C: Depending on the facility's policies, some items may be eligible for reprocessing or recycling. However, any countable items should remain in the room until the procedure is finished and all counts are complete.

61. B: Any PPE that is visibly soiled should be changed in between cases. If not visibly soiled, it is not necessary to change hair covers, shoe covers, or scrubs in between cases.

62. A: In the event of a spill during the case, the circulator should clean the spill as appropriate. Depending on the type of spill, this may require additional personnel or equipment. The circulator should refer to the OSHA manual if there are any questions about how the spill should be handled. The spill should be cleaned as soon as possible to ensure the OR remains a safe environment for other staff members.

63. B: Preventive maintenance is an important process to ensure equipment is available and operable when it is needed for procedures. However, some of this equipment may be in high demand. When preparing for preventive maintenance, the team should review the upcoming surgical schedule to see how the equipment's unavailability may impact future cases. Cases may need to be postponed if spare or loaner equipment is not available.

64. D: The implant paperwork from the manufacturer should be completed and returned to the manufacturer. In the event of a recall, the manufacturer may need to contact the patients with the recalled implant. The circulator should also document the necessary details of the implant in the patient's medical record.

65. A: It should be included in the implant documentation. The fluid used for tissue reconstitution should be sterile fluid that has not already been used during the procedure. The circulator should document the fluid being used for reconstitution as part of the implant record, and this documentation should include the lot number and expiration date of the fluid that has been confirmed with the scrubbed personnel preparing the tissue.

66. C: A tear in the paper count sheet would not indicate the possibility of contamination of a sterile tray. However, moisture in the outer pan or a hole in the paper filter may indicate that the instrument tray's sterility has been compromised. Further, the sterile indicator in the tray should be confirmed as positive prior to placing the instruments on the sterile field.

67. A: Equipment needs for cases should be reviewed and confirmed prior to the day of surgery. If the equipment is unavailable, this may result in the case needing to be postponed or canceled. This should be avoided on the day of surgery whenever possible to prevent operational inefficiencies and inconvenience to the patient.

68. D: In order to maintain professional accountability, the nursing staff should constantly monitor for changes to regulatory guidelines and recommendations. Subscribing to journals is a great way to stay informed of these changes. If the changes contradict the facility's policies or procedures, the nurse should have their manager to review the impact.

69. B: People in caregiving professions, such as nursing or social work, are at high risk of developing compassion fatigue. Compassion fatigue is a type of emotional exhaustion that occurs after repeat exposure to someone else's physical, emotional, or mental trauma. While perioperative nurses have physically demanding roles that can lead to lower back issues, lumbar strains are a type of physical occupational hazard, not a psychosocial one. Therefore, Choice *A* can be eliminated. Codependency is a psychosocial issue that presents itself in personal relationships, such as romantic or familial ones. It is not typically associated with operating room hazards, so Choice *C* can be eliminated. Needle sticks are a biological hazard; they occur if a provider accidentally sticks themselves with a sharp item that may contain bodily fluids from a patient. While the stress of this can cause psychological distress, it is not primarily characterized as a psychosocial issue, so Choice *D* can be eliminated.

70. C: The presence of even small quantities of alcohol in the system can cause significant interactions with anesthesia that is administered for surgical procedures. Prior recommendations to abstain for twenty-four hours prior to surgery are considered outdated; healthcare providers now recommend abstaining from alcohol for at least forty-eight hours prior to surgery, with longer abstinence periods possibly being more beneficial for the patient. Alcohol is linked with worse surgical outcomes and longer post-op recovery times. It is recommended that patients take extra good care of their health prior to surgery, including moderate or low-impact exercise (depending on the type of procedure) and extra rest, so Choices *A* and *B* can be eliminated. Group activities are not likely to hinder surgical outcomes; in fact, positive social events and having a sense of community alongside a complex medical intervention can support better recovery. Choice *D* is incorrect.

71. A: The Patient Protection and Affordable Care Act makes it illegal for health insurance companies to change or cancel someone's health insurance plan due to a pre-existing condition or new illness. The Consolidated Omnibus Budget Reconciliation Act allows some employees to maintain prior job-sponsored health insurance plans in select instances, primarily related to job loss. This does not apply to Bram, so Choice *B* can be eliminated. The Health Insurance Portability and Accountability Act allows someone to have employer-sponsored health insurance in the event of job loss or job change that results in health insurance loss, even if they have a pre-existing condition. Bram has not lost or changed his job or health insurance coverage, so this does not apply. Choice *C* can be eliminated. The Americans with Disabilities Act protects citizens with documented disabilities from any type of exclusionary activities. This context does not pertain to Bram, so Choice *D* can be eliminated.

72. D: Physicians and nurses involved in surgery have over twice the rate of musculoskeletal injuries than the general population; this is believed to be due to the highly physical nature of surgical work, including operating for long periods of time in abnormal or unnatural postures. Ergonomics is an important aspect of maintaining occupational health for people who work in surgery. While medical providers tend to have higher rates of burnout than other professions, it is not twice the rate of the population in general; therefore, Choice *A* can be eliminated. Rates of chronic diseases such as heart disease and being overweight or obese are rising in healthcare workers; however, they still tend to be less in these workers than in the general population. Therefore, Choices *B* and *C* are incorrect.

73. C: Surgical skin prep is a pre-operative process in which the surgical sites on the patient's skin are cleaned of any foreign bodies and microbes that could cause infection. As all surgical sites are open wounds, asepsis is a critical preparation point of surgery. This process does not necessarily affect how a patient feels about surgery, so Choice *A* can be eliminated. Tearing of the skin is not related to how sterile the skin surface is, but rather surgical precision and subjective health factors of the patient, so Choice *B* can be eliminated. Adverse anesthetic outcomes normally occur due to administration or patient reaction. While infection at the anesthesia site could be considered an adverse outcome, the primary goal of skin prep even at the site of anesthesia administration is to prevent infection. Therefore, Choice *D* can be eliminated.

74. B: Any sealed sterile items that need to be added to a sterile field should be opened with the package facing away from the handler. The handler should hold the bottom of the package with one hand and peel the seal back from the farthest corner, ensuring that there is no contact with the packaged items. The sterile item should be gently shaken out of the container at an angle so that it can drop into the sterile field without contact and be given a perimeter of one inch from any other materials. All items in the sterile field should be prepped for use and the surgeon should not need to open any items during surgery itself; therefore, Choice *A* can be eliminated. A sterile item should not be placed into any other container between its own packaging and transport to the sterile field, so Choice *C* is incorrect. The handler should not come into contact with the sterile item at all; wiping it with an antiseptic wipe can inadvertently introduce microbes from the handler's skin. Choice *D* can be eliminated.

75. C: Class III wounds are those in which the wound is exposed to external contamination at the time of formation. In Choice *C*, the nail causes the wound and also introduces an external vector for pathogens. A corneal scratch is relatively minor, and the contact lens would have been sterile. This is most likely to be classified as a "clean" wound, or a Class I wound, so Choice *A* is incorrect. Any wound exposed to fecal matter is a Class IV, or dirty-contaminated wound.

This is the case even if it is due to a controlled surgical operation. Choice *B* falls into this category and can be eliminated. An endoscopic surgery is a controlled site that is kept as sterile as possible; however, the esophagus is exposed to many microbes that live in the gut. Therefore, it is at a higher risk of wound infection and is known as a Class II wound, or a clean-contaminated wound. These classification factors signify the infection risk for a wound, with Class I wounds having the lowest risk for infection. However, patient factors also contribute to infection risk (e.g., smokers are at higher risk for wound infection even in seemingly minor wounds). Choice *D* is incorrect.

Communication and Documentation

1. D: Each of these settings is an example of a location in which the perioperative interview may take place. Perioperative interviews are likely to take place days or weeks in advance of the procedure in a setting other than an operating room.

2. C: The nurse interviewing the patient should document the potential risk factors that are associated with the patient not having transportation. Also, the nurse should notify the surgeon that the patient is currently without transportation following the procedure. The nurse may need to also contact a social worker to identify other viable options to get the patient home safely following the procedure. The nurse may also prepare to reschedule.

3. A: Clinical information technology centers on a set of clinical tasks, instruments, equipment, and imaging. The other options listed are mainly associated with health care information technology, which has a broader base of processes and functions such as laboratory, pharmacy, and admissions.

4. C: Information technology provides for advancement in the perioperative setting. It is an important asset that allows for efficiency and cost savings and improves the overall quality of care.

5. B: The nurse could receive a suspension or lose her job, and the facility could also face a significant fine. This is the best answer, as HIPAA violations are costly for the violator and organization associated with the violation.

6. A: Perioperative checklists provide a method to track and manage the execution of policies and procedures that are in place within a perioperative department.

7. C: The Patient Safety and Quality Improvement Act (PSQIA) leaves it up to organizations to self-report errors without being subject to HIPAA violations; all patient information is kept confidential. HIPAA is a patient privacy act that aims to keep patient health information private. FAFSA is a student aid form. ADA refers to the Americans with Disabilities Act, which isn't relevant here.

8. A: Patients are most susceptible to adverse effects in their care or health status during or after a transition in staffing, especially if there's inadequate communication between transitioning members regarding the patient's condition and needs. The other situations are not necessarily contexts that can be disadvantageous for the patient.

9. C: CUS stands for Concerned, Uncomfortable, and Safety; this technique allows a staff member to indicate concern about the patient's vital signs, if they are uncomfortable regarding the plan for the patient, or if there's a safety concern. Jonah addresses all of these when he states that the patient has been showing questionable health signs and that he feels it's not safe or acceptable to discharge the patient. The SBAR and I PASS the BATON techniques refer to transition steps between team members that occur whether or not extra concern should be shown regarding the patient. TeamSTEPPS refer to communication techniques that nurses can utilize with interdisciplinary care providers.

10. B: The pre-operative interview allows the nurse to discuss the patient's medical and health history (to prepare necessary equipment, medication, and personnel for the procedure) and the operative procedure in depth with the patient. Patient finances, case studies, and behaviors that contributed to the need for the procedure aren't usually discussed during the pre-operative process, as this can cause anxiety, guilt, shame, and other negative feelings for the patient. The pre-operative interview is meant to be an informative and soothing process.

11. B: Busy clinical settings often require staff members to engage with multiple tasks and multiple patients. This can commonly lead to inadequate hand-offs. Physical disabilities and colleague absences aren't common causes of communication barriers in a clinical setting.

12. A: The use of mobile work stations, electronic medical records, integrated clinic and pharmacy systems, and patient portal systems all indicate a medical organization that's fully utilizing healthcare information technology. The online practices illustrated in the case are helping the providers access, document, and maintain patient files more efficiently. The case also illustrates how online systems allow an interdisciplinary team to work together to deliver treatment that the patient needs. Paper charting systems aren't relevant to this case. The proximity of the pharmacy and the demeanor of the pharmacist is a benefit for the patient, but these aren't recurring themes presented in the case.

13. C: Posting on social media about a case and identifying personal information violates HIPAA, which aims to protect patient privacy and health information. The other options aren't relevant.

14. D: While perioperative education is linked to better overall outcomes for the patient upon discharge, there are no guarantees that the patient's post-discharge care will be problem-free. The other options listed are benefits of perioperative education.

15. A: Many nurses may find themselves in (or actively seek out) non-clinical office tasks such as project management, business analyses (such as operational improvements), and software development. This can be a rewarding addition to the work day for those who are interested in these topics. Or, it may simply be a need of the clinic. Nurses generally won't oversee excessive clean-up for the clinic. Choices *C* and *D* may be tasks that nurses undertake, but both are still clinical responsibilities.

16. D: There are a number of influential things that may impact the hand-off process for perioperative staff, including establishing and maintaining an environment that runs smoothly. This drive to keep things running smoothly can ultimately prove distracting during a hand-off.

17. C: A good hand-off provides information that is accurate, clear, and specific. A good hand-off allows for open discussion between the perioperative nurse providing information about the patient and the nurse who is receiving the patient. Poor communication during a hand-off increases the risk for errors and poor patient outcomes.

18. B: Patients or families who do not understand postoperative care needs for the patient may create an atmosphere of risk for poor patient outcomes. The patient or family needs to have a strong understanding of postoperative care needs prior to surgery and again prior to discharge. While the other answers are "good-to-know" information, the surgeon has to be made aware of details that indicate risk for the patient.

19. C: Children may benefit from exposure to the perioperative environment and terminology in the days or weeks preceding surgery to reduce anxiety. Nurses should show empathy and prepare themselves to not only answer the questions of the children, but also answer the questions of the parents.

20. D: Patient education is critical to patient outcomes during the postoperative period. Patients who fully understand what to expect before, during, and after a procedure tend to recover faster, thus reducing their hospital stay or recovery time. Also, they exhibit more satisfaction because they understand what is happening and do not require as much pain medication.

21. A: Gaps in knowledge/understanding is the best answer. Perioperative staff should continuously monitor the patient's level of understanding when education is provided the same day instead of the days following surgery.

22. C: Instruments from an external source should be resterilized before use to ensure that sterility parameters have been met. It should not be assumed that items remain sterile during transit from an outside source. Items should be tracked or logged upon arrival; however, sterility is the most important component to consider prior to use.

23. A: A major benefit of an electronic health record is that it can be easily accessed by multiple providers, which increases access to coordinated, interdisciplinary care for patients, improves quality of care, and reduces medical errors. Additionally, patients can access their medical records easily, which can improve patient satisfaction. At this time, types of health records used vary by country, and accessing one's record in a different country will likely require additional steps. Therefore, Choice *B* can be eliminated. Training is extensive, as users need to be trained on data input, data management, security, and other administrative protocols, so Choice *C* can be eliminated. Rural facilities have had a harder time with the implementation and adoption of electronic health record systems, due to lower tech literacy in patient populations and limited tech and internet availability, therefore, Choice *D* can be eliminated.

24. D: Prior authorization is a process that takes place before a medical procedure is performed. In this process, a patient and their healthcare provider receive approval for payment from the patient's health insurance provider (if applicable) for the procedure. This process should never occur after the procedure has been performed, unless the patient is prepared to pay out-of-pocket. Infection prevention is a critical component of patient discharge to avoid readmittance, so Choice *A* can be eliminated. When a patient has a medical procedure, their discharge instruction should include permission for whether the patient can drive themselves home. If they cannot, there should be a documented plan for how they will leave the medical facility and go home. Therefore, Choice *B* can be eliminated. Discharge information also includes educational information (and sometimes pharmaceutical counseling) about any medications the patient will need to use after a medical procedure, so Choice *D* can be eliminated.

25. C: In healthcare, downtime refers to periods when the electronic medical record/electronic health record and/or other clinical software critical for clinical and administrative operations stop working or are inaccessible. This can occur due to technology issues such as internet outages, software problems, or hardware concerns; they can also result from natural disasters and mass casualty events when patient volume becomes too high for electronic systems to be used efficiently. For example, in mass casualty events, patients often end up being seen in in makeshift areas where computers and lab equipment are not available. During downtime periods, patient access to care is often compromised. For example, providers may not be able to use their normal systems to order labs or other medical interventions, and patients typically cannot access their own medical records and documents. Therefore, Choice *A* can be eliminated. While triage may be used during times of natural disaster, mass casualty events, or other instances of overcapacity, this process is typically not implemented due to internet outages and software glitches, so Choice *B* can be eliminated. An increase in tetanus vaccinations is not directly linked to any of the listed causes, so Choice *D* is incorrect.

Infection Prevention and Control

1. B: Sterile water should be used to irrigate channels and flush debris from instruments. Saline should not be utilized for this process because it can cause mineral deposits to form. Tap water can cause contamination, and lactated Ringer's solution is not commonly used to keep instruments moist.

2. C: The best practice is to keep sterilization records on file for a minimum of three years.

3. C: High-level disinfectants are regulated by the FDA, while low- and intermediate-level disinfectants are regulated by the Environmental Protection Agency (EPA).

4. A: Any instrument that comes in contact with a component of the vascular system (such as the lungs) or sterile tissue is considered a critical item. Semicritical items are those that come in contact with mucous membranes. Noncritical items don't make contact with any part of the body other than unbroken skin. Disinfecting agents don't determine the critical level that items fall under on the Spaulding Classification System.

5. D: 1 in 1,000,000. Proper sterilization of equipment is essential because it significantly reduces microorganism survival rate.

6. B: Blood pressure cuffs only come in contact with unbroken skin, making it a noncritical item. Critical items are those that come in contact with the vascular system or sterile tissue. Blood pressure cuffs can be reliable in nature and used as a monitoring tool, but these answers don't relate to the Spaulding Classification System.

7. B: Sodium hypochlorite is the only commonly used disinfecting agent that possesses all of the listed characteristics. Sodium peroxide is a cleaning agent commonly found in laundry detergents and other household cleaning items but is typically not used in medical settings. Formaldehyde and hydrogen peroxide don't possess all the qualities listed, though they're commonly used in medical settings.

8. B: Steam sterilization possesses all of the listed qualities and is commonly used to clean instruments and other items in hospital settings. Wiping with a cloth isn't considered a sterile cleaning method. Infrared sterilization isn't used in healthcare settings. Freeze-motivated sterilization isn't a real sterilization method.

9. A: When a sterile package falls on the floor, is exposed to water or extreme temperatures, is ripped or damaged, or is stored longer than its expiration date, it shouldn't be used in a medical procedure.

10. C: This isn't a common protocol employed by medical organization, though the other three methods listed are commonly employed strategies for preventing cross-contamination.

11. A: All chemotherapy orders must be written orders received from a physician on the proper form. Even if scheduling is available, the patient is prepared, the physician is present, and Aria feels comfortable performing the procedure, chemotherapy administration cannot occur without the written physician orders.

12. D: This is the first step for any externally sourced instrument to ensure its sterilization and log that it came from an external source. While a physician will likely inspect the item before use and it may be stored for a few days, these aren't usually the first steps that occur. Representatives from the respective manufacturing company aren't normally present when items are transported or loaned.

13. C: A dry, temperature-controlled room that has limited staff access. In addition to these qualities, shelving that isn't adjacent to the floor, ceiling, or walls is also preferable. The other qualities listed aren't preferable; they can actually be harmful for the sterilization and safety of the instruments.

14. C: All of the answer choices are types of standard precautions, but research has shown that proper hand hygiene using soap and water or alcohol-based hand rub (if appropriate) is the best way to prevent the spread of germs.

15. B: The classic signs of infection are redness, heat, and swelling. If the wound is cool to the touch but appears normal otherwise, that is not suggestive of a developing infection. It may be a sign of decreased blood flow to the site, but the nurse should do a full assessment before jumping to that conclusion.

16. C: The incubation period is the point in time where the organism has already invaded the person's body through a portal of entry, is multiplying, and is getting ready to manifest the first symptoms of infection. The colonization occurs right after entry into the body where the organism takes up residence in the host and prepares to multiply. The prodromal period is when the person develops general signs or symptoms (such as fatigue, headache, fever, etc.) before developing more specific signs and symptoms that help point towards a diagnosis. The convalescent period is when the person is recovering from the illness.

17. C: The first piece of personal protective equipment the nurse should don is a gown, Choice *C*. Choice *A*, gloves, are donned next, followed by Choice *B*, mask, and ultimately, Choice *D*, goggles, are donned last. The nurse must follow this sequence to ensure protection against infection transmission.

18. D: Personal protective equipment (PPE) must be removed at the patient's doorway. In addition, it would also be appropriate to remove PPE just outside the patient's room. PPE must not be removed at the nursing station, Choice *A*, at the bedside, Choice *B*, or in the patient's bathroom, Choice *C*, as these occurrences would put infection control and safety at risk.

19. C: Gloves and a disposable mask are all that are required for droplet precaution; however, additional PPE may be used if desiring extra protection. The key word in this question is *minimum.* Choice *A* is not correct because an N-95 mask is not required. Choice *D* is not correct because sterile gloves are not needed, and eyewear is optional. Choice *B* would give the most coverage for protection, but it is not the minimum PPE required.

20. B: Perioperative inoculation occurs around the time of surgery and happens most frequently in joint replacement surgery. Although it could be considered a post op infection, its cause is perioperative and not post-operative. Infectious arthritis, a joint infection, is not exclusively the result of surgery.

21. D: Choice *D* indicates the appropriate level of infection control to reduce the risk of transmission for a patient diagnosed with active tuberculosis. Choices *A*, *B*, and *C* would not provide enough protection in reducing this risk. Tuberculosis is an airborne disease; therefore, transmission of the bacillus, mycobacterium tuberculosis, must be minimized.

22. A. Terminal cleaning should occur daily, or every 24 hours, to ensure proper decontamination of the operating room. Terminal cleaning involves evaluation of ventilation systems, washing equipment and furniture, and wet vacuuming the floors.

23. B. A scalpel requires sterilization. Scalpels are surgical instruments that come into contact with sterile tissues and can transmit microorganisms if not sterilized properly.

24. C. Single-use items are intended to remain packaged until they are used. Once the package has been opened, whether intentionally or accidentally, the item must be used or discarded. Single-use items are not intended to be reused, disinfected, or sterilized.

25. B. Sterilization procedures are monitored and evaluated by mechanical, chemical, and biological indicators. Mechanical indicators monitor the cycle time, pressure, and temperature of steam sterilization. Chemical monitors use sensitive tabs, tapes or strips that change color when they are exposed to temperature changes. Biological monitors use spores to assess the effectiveness of the sterilizer in killing resistant microorganisms. Sterilization procedures are not monitored and evaluated by clinical indicators, making Choice *B* the only incorrect answer.

26. C. A genital swab is considered a biohazard specimen. Biohazard materials are potentially infectious and must be appropriately labeled. A red bag designates the specimen as a biohazard.

27. D. A scalpel is considered a sharp instrument and should be disposed of in an appropriate sharps container. Disposing of sharps in a biohazard bag can increase the risk of a penetrating injury.

28. C. A lead apron protects OR personnel from exposure to radiation. Cumulative non-protected exposure to radiation can lead to cell mutations and cancer.

29. A. The Bowie-Dick test is a chemical monitoring tool used to ensure that air is removed effectively from the sterilization chamber of a dynamic-air-removal system. A uniform color change on the test sheet indicates a successful result.

30. B. Sterile packages should not be stacked on top of each other. Packages should have enough air circulation from all angles to prevent temperature changes.

31. D. Tagging the package or using barcode technology upon arrival at the facility ensures tracking throughout the course of initial processing, use, and decontamination postoperatively.

32. C. A scrub station is designated as a restricted zone. A mask must be applied to prevent contamination of surfaces through oral and nasal secretions.

33. B: Room turnover is a process that entails cleaning the room after one patient is discharged and preparing it for the next patient. It involves sterilizing high-touch areas, changing bed linens, removing waste products and trash from the prior patient out of the room, sweeping and mopping floors, and ensuring all tools are available and prepped for the next patient. This is required to ensure patient safety and hygiene. While some surgical teams may have janitorial support, this is not always the case, and team members should be prepared to clean and sanitize as needed.

The surgical team is not responsible for managing financial counseling, such as insurance reimbursement or payment plans, for the family. Medical facilities generally have an administrative team member who supports the patient with this aspect prior to the procedure. Therefore, Choice *A* can be eliminated. At this time, no federal requirement for lunch breaks exists; state laws vary greatly. Therefore, staggered lunch times for the team are not a requirement and Choice *C* is incorrect. The surgery team typically would not be responsible for administrative responsibilities such as software updates. Even if they were, it would be unlikely that they would manage these in between emergency cases; therefore, Choice *D* can be eliminated.

34. B: Circulating nurses serve a vital role on the surgery team. Circulating nurses are responsible for patient advocacy, communicating information between the operating room and the other parts of the hospital, and supporting with tasks such as room and equipment preparation. While circulating nurses may help ensure that sterile equipment is provided in a timely and safe manner to the surgeon, they are not required to formally scrub in and carry out sterile techniques and processes during the actual surgery. This is the job of the scrub nurse, who works as an immediate assistant to the surgeon for hands-on tasks. Therefore, Choice *A* can be eliminated. A nurse anesthetist primarily supports with administering anesthesia to the patient, so Choice *C* is incorrect. A sterile compounding technician typically works in a pharmacy to make drugs that require sterile techniques and would not be present in an operating room. Choice *D* can be eliminated.

35. A: Restricted zones require fully sterile, scrubbed-in apparel to prevent exposure risks. Not only do these zones require shoe covers, but they also require approved scrubs, masks, and head and hair coverings. Some examples of restricted zones include the operating room and the newborn intensive care unit. Semi-restricted zones do have some stringent requirements, such as approved scrubs and head and hair coverings, but do not generally require shoe covers or masks. Examples of these may include a lab imaging area or food preparation area. Therefore, Choices *B* and *D* can be eliminated. Unrestricted areas are accessible by the general population and street clothes are permitted. Examples include the waiting room and public restroom in the facility. Choice *C* is therefore incorrect.

36. D: Washing hands with soap and water using evidence-based techniques (e.g., cleaning for at least twenty seconds, ensuring all surface areas are covered with soap, vigorous scrubbing) is the gold standard for hand hygiene; however, using an alcohol-based hand sanitizer can be effective in low-risk contexts. Providers should perform hand hygiene prior to putting gloves on; using hand sanitizer according to evidence-based techniques (e.g., covering all surface areas with the sanitizer and allowing contact and drying for twenty seconds) is an effective method for maintaining hand hygiene upon glove removal. A paper cut on one's hand exposes bodily fluids. It should be washed with soap and water and then bandaged to avoid exposing others, so Choice *A* can be eliminated. Hand-washing should occur after using the restroom and after touching fungal spores, as there is a high risk of contamination from pathogens that could seriously harm a patient. Therefore, Choices *B* and *C* can both be eliminated.

Emergency Situations

1. C: Malignant hyperthermia. This condition can occur in surgery, and patients can overheat to a life-threatening temperature. The other conditions are less likely to happen during a surgical procedure, as most patients will be anesthetized; regardless, they wouldn't be characterized by these symptoms.

2. B: Administer dantrolene at a dose of 2.5 mg/kg. This will produce the fastest recovery for the patient and is the safest method to undertake in a surgical setting. Cooling the patient through manual, external modalities is usually not ideal in the operating room. The other options listed aren't relevant.

3. D: These items are common allergens that can cause life-threatening allergic reactions including anaphylaxis (which can ultimately result in suffocation and death). It's vital to make sure all patient allergies are known and accommodated for to the best of the medical team's abilities.

4. B: The heart is often indirectly affected by a number of emergency contexts. The way some primary critical conditions, such as malignant hyperthermia, impact the body almost always impact the functioning of the cardiac muscle as well. Patients may initially experience a primary condition that ultimately results in cardiac arrest. The other options are uncommon secondary conditions that occur during emergencies.

5. A: Patients susceptible to malignant hyperthermia during surgical procedures include those with a prior history of anesthesia complications. Dantrolene should be kept on hand to mitigate any complications that arise. The surgery outcome won't necessarily be affected if the team is prepared.

6. C: The patient's insurance status and paperwork are not responsibilities that the circulator handles. The circulator primarily manages tasks related to emergency situations, team workflow and management, and materials preparation.

7. A: These three components create "the fire triangle." An oxidizer can be an agent like an oxygen tank. An ignition source includes triggers like lasers or electric units. Items that can fuel a blaze include alcohol wipes, large pieces of cloth, or towels. These are all common items in an operating room, unlike the items listed in Choices *B* or *C*. Surgical fires also don't often occur from poor personnel awareness.

8. A: Most organization categorizes emergencies by color code. For example, many hospitals use "Code Red" to indicate a fire outbreak and "Code Orange" to indicate disaster casualties.

9. B: Epinephrine is the most common treatment for patients suffering a severe allergic response. Augmentin and amoxicillin are penicillin-oriented drugs and can often make an allergic reaction worse. Electroshock therapy isn't used to treat allergies.

10. B: All medical facilities should have written, comprehensive disaster plans that can be consulted to adequately prepare and implement procedures in the event of a natural disaster or environmental threat. In this case, reviewing the hospital's flood insurance policy isn't necessary for the staff, and a fire drill is unlikely to occur during a hurricane. Ride-sharing credits aren't relevant to this case.

11. C: Smoke evacuators are used in the operating room when the team is performing a procedure that could result in noxious fumes, such as when conducting surgery using lasers. This prevents noxious fume inhalation by the patient and by healthcare personnel. The other items listed aren't used for this purpose.

12. B: Crash carts are most commonly used for patients experiencing cardiac arrest, regardless as to their demographics. They contain tools such as bag valve masks, defibrillators, and medications, which are useful in emergency situations. Patients in cardiac arrest typically need comprehensive attention within minutes to survive, and the crash cart allows all of the necessary equipment and medication to be readily available.

13. A: A scrub technician often works with the circulating nurse; this role ensures the operating room is clean and orderly, and all equipment and supplies are available and ready to use.

14. C: Electrocautery pencils can come into contact with alcohol-based equipment (such as wipes) or other liquids and cause fires. Scalpels and smoke evacuators are unlikely to cause fires. Heating pads aren't typically used in surgical procedures.

15. B: As the team hasn't begun the procedure, it's best to get to safety and bring the necessary equipment with them. They should avoid operating in an unsafe location at all costs and shouldn't abandon each other or the patient. Even if they had begun the procedure, it would be best to try and evacuate. In this instance, the surgical wound would need to be tended to prior to transport.

16. C: The riskiest component of a laparoscope is its cord, which can cause fires. The other options aren't applicable or true.

17. D: Latex allergies are relatively common and often hereditary. As most organizations use latex gloves and materials unless an allergy is known, complications can result for patients who are allergic to latex. Knowing whether the patient or any of the patient's family members have allergies to latex or bananas allows the circulating nurse and surgical team to properly prepare for the procedure.

18. B: The diuretic reduces blood volume, and the ACE inhibitor reduces SVR by interfering with the RAAS. A CCB works by increasing myocardial contractility; therefore, Choice *A* is incorrect. Choice *C* is incorrect because an ARB reduces systemic vascular resistance, but morphine is used to treat pain. Choice *D* is also incorrect because a beta-blocker increases myocardial contractility.

19. D: An INR of 3.5 is elevated and will cause bleeding complications if thrombolytic therapy is initiated before the INR returns to the normal level of less than or equal to 1.1.

20. D: Hypoventilation and hypoxia are the primary causes of death in chest trauma. Assessing oxygenation and preparing for placement of a chest drain to alleviate a possible hemothorax or pneumothorax are the correct first actions. Pain medication is secondary to ensuring airway, breathing, and circulation. A medical history is important, but it is secondary to the lifesaving interventions.

21. C: An interim chain of command provides a hierarchy of order for staff to follow in the event of a regional emergency. It may involve people from sister facilities or other first response agencies. A documented and recognized chain of command specific to this context minimizes the risks from communication issues or new processes during a vulnerable time. Hurricane evacuation plans may be important for coastal facilities where hurricanes are likely, but they are not necessary for all facilities (e.g., a Midwestern location) and could be a waste of time and resources. Therefore, Choice *A* can be eliminated. A temporary morgue is a waste of cost and space until it is actually needed, so Choice *B* can be eliminated. While hospitals may want to have a secure plan for procuring extra PPE if the need arises, storing them unnecessarily can also be a waste of money and storage space; therefore, Choice *D* can be eliminated.

22. D: Failed intubation occurs when something significant is obstructing the airway of a patient in need. Failed intubation is most likely to occur in patients who have suffered a head, neck, face, or dental injury; have short or thick necks; are obese; have dentures; or are continuously asphyxiating (e.g., due to the presence of blood). After three attempts to intubate a patient, another form of assisted ventilation should be pursued. Medical suction is a process that is often required in patients who cannot be intubated, but it is a technique and not a type of emergency condition; therefore, Choice *A* is incorrect. A heart attack is a medical emergency but is not especially correlated with failed intubation, so Choice *B* can also be eliminated. A blown vein occurs most often after a needle injury to the vein. These are not usually major events and can heal on their own. Regardless, they are not related to intubation, so Choice *D* can be eliminated.

23. A: Due to the nature of the patient's injury and the symptoms he is presenting, the patient should be examined for bleeding in the brain, which can quickly progress to a stroke or other event that can cause long-lasting disability. With early intervention, the long-term effects can be reduced or prevented. Meningitis is an infection of the brain that presents with fever and musculoskeletal pain, especially in the neck. The patient is not showing these specific symptoms or any indication that he was exposed to a pathogen that could cause this condition, so it does not seem like a likely cause of the other neurological symptoms he is showing. Choice *B* can be eliminated. While the patient may have musculoskeletal injury from the fall, it is more important to check for brain bleeding and neurological injuries first to avoid irreparable, systemic damage; therefore, Choice *C* can be eliminated. Dementia occurs over a prolonged period of time before a diagnosis is formally made; it is not typically diagnosed immediately after an acute injury; therefore, Choice *D* is incorrect.

Professional Accountabilities

1. A: If the circulator observes actions or behaviors that undermine a culture of safety, the circulator should speak up and escalate as needed regardless of the team member's role or credentials. As the patient advocate, the circulator must ensure that these behaviors are addressed.

2. C: Assume the edge of the sterile table has been contaminated. If another team member thinks the sterile field has been contaminated, the circulator should assume that the sterility has been compromised and respond accordingly. Even if the circulator or other team members did not witness the reported event, the circulator should err on the side of caution and assume the field was contaminated.

3. B: Nurses should participate in professional development activities whenever possible, balancing time and job demands. These activities may be within the facility or outside the organization. This participation helps maintain professional accountability.

4. B: Ask the charge nurse if the equipment representative is available for assistance. If the staff members are asked to use a piece of equipment that they have not been trained on, they should inform the surgeon that they have not received training or used the equipment before. If the representative for the equipment or other trained team member is available, they may be able to guide the staff in first-time use of the equipment. The staff should not assume that the surgeon is capable of preparing or assembling the device. Further, the circulator should exhaust all available options for assistance and avoid refusing to open the item.

5. D: The staff should search for the needle even though it is very small. If the count is incorrect because of a missing small needle, the staff should follow the facility's policy and procedure. Depending on the size of the needle, an x-ray may not be required because it may not be detectable by x-ray. The surgeon should be informed of the incorrect count and made aware of the needle size and follow-up activities. Even though the needle may be small, the staff should still search the floor and sterile field for the missing needle.

6. B: All types of adverse events should be reported as soon as reasonably possible, even if the nurse's shift extends into overtime. Timely reporting of events ensures that necessary details are not omitted or forgotten. The nurse should follow the facility's policies and procedures for event reporting, which may include documentation in an internal tracking system. The nurse should document the appropriate information in the patient's medical record, but there may be potentially causative details that are not appropriate in the patient's medical record. The nurse should review the report and documentation with their supervisor or manager.

7. B: Nurses across disciplines are held accountable to the standards and guidelines established by the Occupational Safety and Health Administration, American Nursing Association, and the specific state guidelines where they are licensed and employed. They aren't held accountable individually to any guidelines of the Food and Drug Administration, the Environmental Protection Agency, the Department of Health and Human Services, or the Centers for Disease Control, making Choices *A*, *C*, and *D* incorrect.

8. B: The Association of perioperative Registered Nurses determines these domains, which are respected due to the organization's leadership in surgical healthcare practices. The CDC, Mayo Clinic, and Johns Hopkins University are all reputable organizations, but they don't have established guidelines for perioperative nurses, making Choices *A*, *C*, and *D* incorrect.

9. A: In surgical cases, all team members are responsible for a specific scope of tasks that helps the team work efficiently and without adverse effects for the team and patient. Nurses should not take on tasks outside of their scope or discipline, even if they feel like it's a task they could handle. Apart from causing disruption in workflow, it could constitute as malpractice in some instances. If Janna truly feels unable to handle the case in a way that wouldn't compromise the patient's safety, she should speak to the team leader about how to proceed, without involving other team members scheduled for the case.

10. A: While these aren't professional opportunities directly involved with delivering patient care, they're invaluable healthcare roles for which nurses, with their wide range of diverse experiences in the field, make excellent candidates. These are tasks meant for nursing individuals that are further along in their careers (rather than students) and aren't jobs that can be completed remotely.

11. C: Positive changes in workflow processes are considered quality improvement projects, as they allow for better healthcare delivery. In this case, hand sanitization is more likely to be efficiently completed, and overall waits and delays are reduced for the clinic as a whole, as a result of Douglas's proposed change. Quality improvements are often small changes that can make a large impact. The other options aren't applicable, as the WHO isn't conducting this type of sanitization initiative, JHCO doesn't implement such changes, and this case isn't understood to be a common dermatology clinic issue.

12. D: The surgical team is most likely to simply discard the package in question and use a new one. It's an informal practice to treat a package as contaminated when any team member, regardless of experience, is concerned about its sterility. This allows nurses to feel empowered and voice concerns during procedures. This practice also avoids conflicts between colleagues.

13. A: The Plan-Do-Study-Act (PDSA) cycle is recommended by the Institute of Healthcare Improvement and the Agency for Healthcare Research and Quality as a simple framework for healthcare providers and administrators to continuously improve processes. A change is selected to test, and the participant or team who is testing the change will plan for the change, do the change, study successes and obstacles related to the change, and act to adopt, abandon, or anchor the change. The DMAIC method (Define, Measure, Analyze, Improve, Control) is similarly used to improve processes, but is more common in manufacturing and business contexts; therefore, Choice *B* can be eliminated. Value-Stream Mapping is another tool for quality improvement, used to show what steps of a process add value to the customer or organization. While it can gather valuable information to determine what kinds of changes could be tested, it does not provide a framework for testing a process change itself, so Choice *C* is incorrect. Lean is a methodology for analyzing how best to maintain or create value while using the least number of resources. It is not related to tests of change, so Choice *D* can be eliminated.

14. C: Out of all categories of nurses, only nurse practitioners can generally prescribe medications. Even nurse practitioners may still require physician approval or signature to do so, depending on the state in which they are licensed and practicing. Registered nurses are not allowed to prescribe medications, so this option is out of their scope of practice. Prescribing medications could jeopardize their job and result in lawsuits. Registered nurses can delegate some nursing responsibilities to medical and nursing assistants, so Choice *A* can be eliminated. Registered Nurses are tasked with inserting catheters for patients who need them and typically cannot delegate this duty, so Choice *B* can be eliminated. Registered Nurses can monitor patient vitals, although they can also ask for support with this task from medical and nursing assistants; therefore, Choice *D* can be eliminated.

15. B: A clinical research nurse focuses on providing nursing responsibilities in a research setting, and often serves a role connecting the research institution with the sample population in a research design. In this setting, Joan is recruiting the sample and completing nursing tasks such as blood draws and a health education intervention, and then sharing data with the person leading this study. There is no indication in this scenario that Joan is pursing a doctorate degree, so Choice *A* is incorrect. There is also no indication in this scenario that Joan is a teaching professor, so Choice *C* can be eliminated. A nurse administrator is responsible for administrative and management tasks pertaining to efficiently running an organization, such as scheduling nursing staff for shifts; Joan clearly has a more clinical role, so Choice *D* can be eliminated.

Index

Nonsteroidal Anti-Inflammatory Drugs (NSAIDS), 22

Dear CFPN Test Taker,

We would like to start by thanking you for purchasing this study guide for your CFPN exam. We hope that we exceeded your expectations.

Our goal in creating this study guide was to cover all of the topics that you will see on the test. We also strove to make our practice questions as similar as possible to what you will encounter on test day. With that being said, if you found something that you feel was not up to your standards, please send us an email and let us know.

We would also like to let you know about other books in our catalog that may interest you.

Adult CCRN

This can be found on Amazon: amazon.com/dp/1637753454

CEN

amazon.com/dp/1637752229

CNOR

amazon.com/dp/1637753004

We have study guides in a wide variety of fields. If the one you are looking for isn't listed above, then try searching for it on Amazon or send us an email.

Thanks Again and Happy Testing!
Product Development Team
info@studyguideteam.com

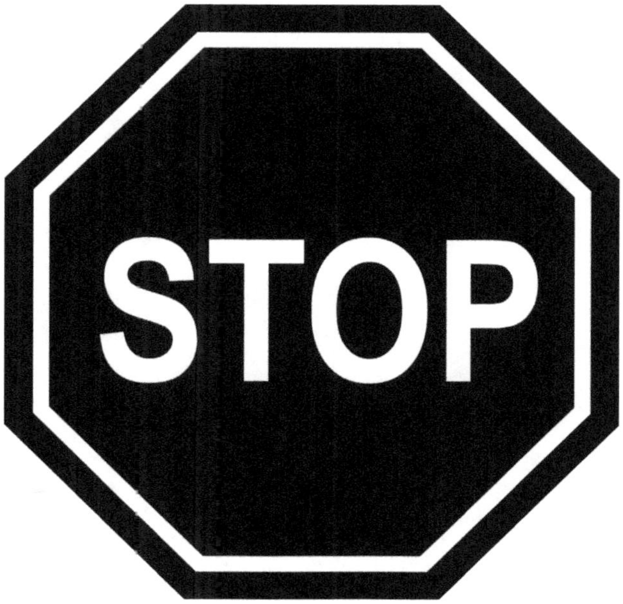

FREE Test Taking Tips Video/DVD Offer

To better serve you, we created videos covering test taking tips that we want to give you for FREE. **These videos cover world-class tips that will help you succeed on your test.**

We just ask that you send us feedback about this product. Please let us know what you thought about it—whether good, bad, or indifferent.

To get your **FREE videos**, you can use the QR code below or email freevideos@studyguideteam.com with "Free Videos" in the subject line and the following information in the body of the email:

a. The title of your product

b. Your product rating on a scale of 1-5, with 5 being the highest

c. Your feedback about the product

If you have any questions or concerns, please don't hesitate to contact us at info@studyguideteam.com.

Thank you!

SCAN HERE

www.ingramcontent.com/pod-product-compliance
Lightning Source LLC
LaVergne TN
LVHW080854070225
803139LV00009B/1688